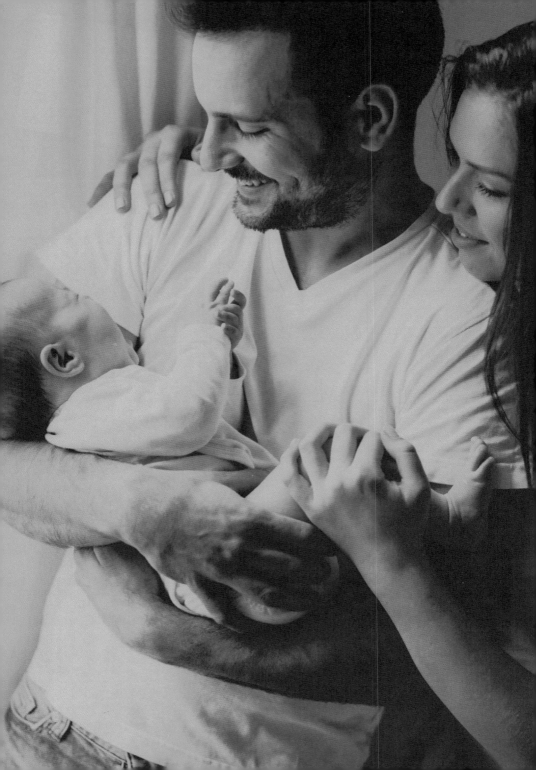

CONTENTS

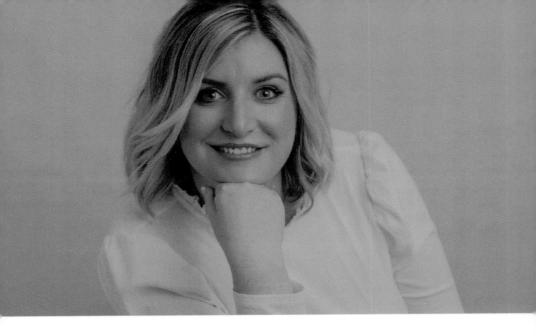

ABOUT THE AUTHOR

I am Lynsey McGillivray, a registered Midwife, Birth Doula, and Hypnobirthing teacher with a passion for transforming perceptions about childbirth. Since 2012, I've been dedicated to guiding individuals through empowering and positive birth experiences.

My journey involves teaching Hypnobirthing through private one-on-one sessions, both in clients' homes and online, connecting with individuals from Saudi Arabia, Brussels, France, Amsterdam, and various other locations. In addition, I facilitate group courses, fostering friendships among expectant parents, and offer an On-demand digital version of my course to enhance accessibility to birth education.

Residing just outside Glasgow, Scotland, with my husband, son, and daughter, I established Born This Way Hypnobirthing to address the prevailing negative mindset surrounding birth. My mission is to dispel fears, instill trust in the birth process, and unveil the incredible, empowering nature of childbirth.

Over the years, I've had the privilege of working with countless individuals, providing them with the knowledge and confidence to approach their unique birth experiences with readiness and positivity, regardless of the unfolding circumstances.

INTRODUCTION

Welcoming your baby into the world is a profound and transformative life event—an experience that should be inherently positive. You deserve not just a good birth but one that resonates as an empowering journey rather than something to endure or survive.

This book aims to revolutionise your perception of childbirth. Recognising the profound connection between your mind and body, it emphasises that if you harbour fears about birth in your mind, your body may resist relaxation and release during labour.

Immersing yourself in positive and authentic birth stories will provide comfort, reassurance, and hopefully ignite a passion for taking charge of your birth experience. Armed with knowledge about the available choices, you can approach childbirth informed and confident.

I am privileged to have the consent of the clients I've worked with to share their unfiltered birth stories. These narratives, written in their own words, offer a genuine glimpse into the diverse experiences of pregnancy and childbirth. They underscore that, irrespective of the birthing method, a sense of being heard, understanding the process, and having autonomy over choices can contribute to an amazing birth experience.

Within the pages of this book, you will encounter a spectrum of birth scenarios, including c-sections, water births, home births, inductions, and assisted deliveries. Whether you are on the journey to conception, currently pregnant, or have experienced childbirth before, this book celebrates the awe-inspiring nature of birth. I am excited for you to discover that, indeed, birth is an extraordinary experience.

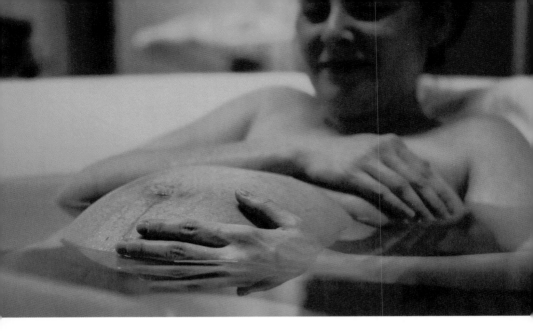

WATER BIRTH

Let's delve into the first birthing method: water birth.

The utilisation of water during labour is gaining popularity owing to its analgesic effects. Water birth is a viable choice in various settings, including home births, midwife-led birthing centres, and select hospital environments.

Contrary to common assumptions, a water birth doesn't solely involve being in a pool. Water can be applied in alternative ways, such as a bath or a targeted hot shower, effectively alleviating sensations.

Key advantages of water birth include:

1. Enhanced Sense of Control:

- The water's buoyancy supports your weight, providing a lighter feeling and promoting comfort.
- The spacious pool allows easy movement, enabling you to intuitively adopt positions that suit your comfort.

2. Relaxing Environment:

- The maintained water temperature at 37 degrees celsius fosters a warm environment for both you and your baby.
- The warmth increases blood circulation, ensuring ample oxygen and blood supply to the uterine muscles for optimal functionality.

3. Perineum Health:

- Increased blood supply to the perineum makes it more elastic, reducing the risk of perineal tears.

While water birth is generally accessible to most, there are circumstances where it might not be recommended. It may not be advisable if you:

- Have been advised to undergo continuous fetal monitoring (unless the birthing setting provides a waterproof monitor).
- Are carrying a pre-term baby (before 37 weeks gestation).
- Have a breech-positioned baby.
- Are expecting multiple pregnancies (twins or triplets).
- Experience vaginal bleeding (difficult to monitor in water).
- Have an infection.
- Have had broken waters for over 24 hours (due to infection risk).
- If the baby has passed meconium.

While water can be used for birthing, some opt to labour in the water and exit for the birthing process. Circumstances may arise where leaving the water is advisable, such as:

- Feeling dizzy or light-headed.
- Having abnormal blood pressure.
- Experiencing bleeding during labour.
- Baby's heartbeat deviates from normal limits.
- Opting to change position or use pain relief.

It's essential to be aware of these considerations to make informed choices for a safe and positive birthing experience.

OLIVIA

I had the most incredibly empowering labour. I absolutely loved the experience of birthing our daughter, so much so that I'd love to do it again and wouldn't change absolutely anything about it. I said immediately after birth that I'd love to relive it all. The midwives caring for me commented that they wished they'd filmed it, as it was so calm and controlled. Start to finish, from my waters breaking to our daughter arriving, was 10 and a half hours in total, only 3 of which were spent in hospital.

Lynsey's private hypnobirthing course was something we'd completed three months earlier. I was keen to invest in birth and be as prepared as we could possibly be. I was a little apprehensive about birth and coping with the pain but also had very strong ideas in my head around avoiding an epidural and wanting a water birth. After a bit of research, Lynsey's classes felt appropriate to gain the relevant information and skills to support. We opted for a private class delivered from the comfort of our home.

My husband was a little unsure going into it all, mainly around what his role was during birth and how he could support me with it, knowing it was me that was birthing our baby and not him. He was easily persuaded to give the classes a go, and it was great to see his mindset shift immediately from the first class. He instantly saw that he had a huge role to play in our baby's birth and was pivotal in supporting and advocating for me. He told me that he could absolutely see why it was important he became involved and informed himself ahead of my labour.

Fast forward to December. Following all of the advice from Lynsey and preparation around breathing techniques, massage, and positioning to ensure my body was ready, my waters went. I woke up at 4 am to the feeling of a trickle of water and knew immediately my waters had gone. I stood up, and there was a Hollywood-style gush, which you don't expect to have. This was it—my husband and I thought! We were incredibly excited to know we'd be meeting our baby girl 9 days sooner than we'd expected from our due date given to us. My body embraced it all with not one bit of fear or tension present.

I went back to bed, and half an hour later, my waves started. I surrendered to them. My body knew exactly what it was doing, and for the past 9 months, was preparing for this day. The waves quickly ramped up in length and intensity. Around 3 hours later, I moved to a bath to give me some relief. My husband ran me one and asked if I'd like a massage or food. I declined and phoned triage to explain my waters had gone, where they reminded me that I should not have them burst beyond 24hrs and should attend triage within 12hrs and a plan made around things. I agreed but was using the BRAIN acronym throughout, knowing we had all the options and didn't feel at all concerned when this was said. I continued in the bath with breathing techniques until the waves increased a notch.

By 9 am, the waves were feeling bigger and longer, so I popped my TENS machine on. It gave the perfect distraction along with swaying my hips from side to side. I was on all fours, leaning over the bed, sofa, or birthing ball during this time. At 10 am, I felt there was a change in my body again, and my husband recognised this too. I felt waves were increasing again, and so I phoned triage back. They advised that it was too soon to go in and I'd likely be sent home. However, they did ask what I'd like to do. I said I was planning on coming anyway, as felt this was appropriate.

It took all my energy between the short gaps of the waves to get dressed and into the car. We left at 10.45 am, and both of us thought I had likely hit the transition stage of labour. I increased the TENS machine level to manage the waves for the 30-minute drive and also used an eye mask to remain in my zone and calm. This wasn't the best position to be sat in during this stage of labour, and I found it quite uncomfortable; however, the breathing techniques supported me greatly.

When we arrived at the hospital, I had an urge to bear down and felt immense pressure in my back passage. I knew then it was likely that I was fully dilated. The walk from the car to triage was an interesting one where I used all my energy and strength to breathe through every wave.

When I arrived at triage, they could tell I was in active labour and swiftly moved me to a bed, asking me to lie down and get ready to be checked. They left me for around 10 minutes; however, I was unable to lie down. I leaned over the bed and was swaying my hips from side to side and going with every wave.

When the midwife came to check me, I explained that I was using hypnobirthing techniques to support me, so it was likely that it might look as if I wasn't as far on as it seemed. She suggested again I lie on the bed to be checked if I could, and she'd also put the baby on a monitor too. My husband reminded me that we'd decided no vaginal exams unless the baby was in distress to ensure my oxytocin levels remained high. He asked me directly if I was sure I wanted this. I agreed as felt it was important to move things forward and ensure I got into the right environment to breathe the baby out. The baby's heart was dipping, which the midwife felt meant it was close to our daughter arriving. She then did a vaginal examination to confirm this. Much to her complete shock and surprise, I was 10cm dilated, and she announced that I was some woman. She could feel the baby's head and told me that I was ready to push.

This was the most euphoric feeling knowing our baby girl was coming so soon. She rushed away, got a birth kit and said I could birth her in triage if required; however, she was keen to get me somewhere more private. I came out of my zone at this point and stopped the hypnobirthing techniques to bring me back into the room to give my body time to get to the midwife unit as I wasn't keen to birth her in triage.

We got in the lift, and the midwife said she had the birth kit there and was gloved up, so was ready to catch the baby. Lying on my back with my legs straight and the bright lights meant it dipped my oxytocin levels. The pressure I felt and urge to push was starting to reduce a little. I was happy with this as I wanted to get into a private space and preferably have that water birth I had in my head.

We arrived at the assisted midwife unit at around 11.45 am, where I remained on the bed for a while before transferring to the foam cubes. I felt I was having a gap between the pushing stage and regaining my energy. I instinctively got onto all fours and swayed my hips from side to side. My husband used tingle touch massage and got my birth playlist on.

There was both a student midwife and midwife present. They remained hands-off throughout and just in the background completing their checks. After a short while, the pool was ready, and they said I could get in if I wished.

This was the only point where I hesitated, as the TENS machine was working so well for me, so I was unsure if removing it might slow things down. The midwives reminded me that I would only know if I tried, and they'd get me out and dried off as quickly as possible if I wasn't happy with it. Between waves, I detached the TENS machine and hopped in. I felt my body sink in and got into an upright, forward, and open position. I swayed side to side with each wave and felt the pressure build. I reminded the team I didn't want coached pushing and would be breathing my baby out.

They respected this to begin with; however, one hour into being in the pool and with me not starting to push, they said they'd have to speak to the Dr and decide on a plan. Babies' vitals and my own were absolutely fine, so there was no reason for any intervention. I reminded them of this and continued to use my BRAIN. The midwife came back and said the Dr was happy to wait and see for another hour. This did feel a little off-putting as a time limit was given to me.

My husband was there by my side offering me water as well as gas and air should I need it and reminded me of trying some down breathing. I only took a few puffs of gas and air when that particular wave felt powerful but didn't need this during every one. He was such a brilliant support for me throughout my labour, gently reminding me of hypnobirthing techniques, encouraging me and just being there.

At 1.30 pm, my body began to surrender to the waves, and I felt this sudden urge to push using down breathing. A change of position was reminded by the midwives, so between each wave, I squatted back then my pulled body forward and pulled against my husband's arm moving slightly upwards. With each wave, my body brought our baby girl gradually and gently lower. I could feel everything slowly open up and her head become lower with each wave. Her heart rate was spot on as was mine during all of this. It was the most exciting thing knowing she was nearly here!

An hour later of down breathing, her head was out and was bobbing up and down in the water with her eyes wide open, looking so calm and serene. The team caring for me could not believe how relaxed she was. With another 2 waves, they thought I'd fully birthed our daughter and suggested that I could lift her out of the water.

It was at that point that I said she wasn't fully out, and it was noted her cord was wrapped around her neck twice as well as around her arm. So when her head came out her arm and hand also did because of the cord. Her heart rate showed no indication of this throughout birth with no dipping or increase seen at all.

She was untangled and with a final down breath, I brought her up between my legs and out of the water. She opened her eyes and calmly breathed away on my chest with her eyes wide open. In my head, I knew there was no loud crying due to the calm and controlled way she'd be brought into the world, but it didn't stop me asking if she was okay, which they said she was.

The midwives all said what a calm and beautiful birth it was and that I'd managed it all so well. I remained in the pool with our baby for a while but was keen to come out to birth my placenta. Everyone helped me out as we'd wanted delayed cord clamping until the cord had completely stopped pulsating. My placenta naturally came away quickly after this, and my midwife checked it all over. She then checked me over for any tears, which there were none. The midwife was surprised at this due to our daughter coming out with her hand up at the side of her face. This meant it was wider than just her head alone coming out. The baby had her first feed at this point, and I got around 2 hours of skin to skin before my husband got a further 45 minutes while I got a shower and changed.

We wrote a birth plan of what we wanted. Every element of it was fulfilled with the only exception being that I arrived further on than we'd put down. I was fully dilated instead of the 7cm we'd noted down.

I felt like superwoman after the birth and still on top of the world from it all. It was such a euphoric moment and will remain with me forever. My body knew exactly what to do, and all that preparation was worth it to have what we feel was the perfect birth for us. I feel so proud of my birth story and both of our shifts in mindset too.

PENELOPE

I believe it's worth mentioning that before undertaking the hypnobirthing course with Lynsey, discussing labour and birth was something I found utterly daunting. This apprehension likely stemmed from numerous birth stories I had heard, read, or seen on television. Positive birth stories seemed scarce, requiring intentional searching.

After trying for just over 2 years, my husband and I finally fell pregnant. We were over the moon, but the anxiety of birth quickly set in. I coped by pushing it to the back of my mind and deciding not to deal with it until much nearer the time (not the best idea, I know). I wouldn't even let myself think about it. Around the 6-month mark, I opened up to a friend who had recently given birth and explained how I was feeling. My friend had a remarkably positive birth experience, which, in my world, was unusual to hear about. She explained that she had done a hypnobirthing course prior and truly believed this was the main contributor to her story.

I did some of my research to see if it was something that suited me, and it all sounded great. But, to be honest, I still had my doubts. That's when I decided to bite the bullet and contact Lynsey. By this point, I didn't have much to lose; I was now 7 months pregnant and still had a lot of anxiety surrounding the birth. After speaking to Lynsey, we chose to go with private Zoom sessions as I felt that I really needed that one-to-one guidance, and due to location, this was the most suitable.

Lynsey also advised having my husband, Shaune, attend the sessions where possible so we could get the absolute most from the course. Before speaking to Lynsey, I honestly thought the course would just be for myself. I am so thankful she recommended Shaune attend as it meant he knew exactly what I was going through and how, as a partner, he could support.

Over the next 4 weeks, Lynsey worked with us to explain exactly what hypnobirthing is all about, the term "hypno" in particular, how the body works, removing the fear, and how Shaune can best support me. Not only were we given one-to-one sessions but also videos and audios to watch and listen to after each session (homework if you like). Being a more visual person, I found the videos especially very oxytocin-releasing to watch and found myself searching for more leading up to the big day.

What I loved the most about the course and what Lynsey went through was that it was all backed by science, studies, and data. It made me truly believe that this is what my body was designed for and that hypnobirthing is an education to help you cope/manage each wave to help make your birth experience a positive one. The course also enables us to be informed about the choices we were making, helping us understand the terms being used and how we wanted to approach each stage for what felt right for us.

At the end of our 4-week course, I had gone from not even being able to think about birth to being excited and ready!

Even before the course, I had always known and loved the idea of having a water birth. But pre-course, I honestly didn't believe it was something I myself could do. How could I when all I had heard, seen, and read about was how much pain I was going to be in and that birth wasn't to be enjoyed or unmedicated but almost injured.

However, after the course, I absolutely believed that this was a birth option for me, and why couldn't we enjoy this after all? It was our daughter's birthday! So we made our wishes known to our midwife and also chose to give birth in a midwife-led unit as the environment and practices seemed to mirror what myself and Shaune wanted for our birth. We wrote out our dream birth and how, if we could choose, it should go. This was something Lynsey suggested we do to help visualise our birth. We loved doing this as it made us excited, almost like planning for a party, which I love to do.

In the early hours of Wednesday morning in June, my contractions started; they were very light and manageable. So I continued with my day, bouncing on my ball, watching Friends, and eating chocolate. I remembered Lynsey said to us that I should be able to continue as normal at the start (this helped pass the time and kept me distracted).

My light contractions lasted until Thursday afternoon before the intensity increased, and I needed some sort of pain relief, which initially came from a hot bath. It took the edge off and helped me focus on my breathing. Later in the night, I switched on the tens machine (another thing recommended by Lynsey). This was a great distraction tool; it didn't take the pain away but did distract me enough to stay focused on my breathing and ride each wave and trust that my body was doing what it needed to do. It got to 1 am Friday morning when I decided that I was ready to go in.

Once we arrived, our midwife had the lights dimmed in the room, calming mood lighting on, and the pool ready, which came as a huge relief and instantly put me at ease. I asked if I could be checked, as I really wanted to know how far I was. I only wanted to do this once, and this was my choice. I felt at the start was best, so I knew where I was at and going, and to my amazement, I was 5 cm! I felt proud and encouraged that everything I was doing was working, and our little girl was on her way.

Once in the pool a few hours later, I asked for some gas and air as I needed a distraction that was more intense than my breathing techniques and Shaune's massages, as good as they were. The gas and air again didn't take the pain away but did distract me enough from the pain and helped me focus back on my breathing, which I honestly believed was my biggest pain relief, along with the noises I was making. I believe I mooed at one point!

I will say that there was a brief moment where I lost it; I began to cry, my breathing focus went, and I started to panic. For a brief moment, I had forgotten everything I had learned and thought I can't do this. I voiced this out loud, which Shaune responded with, "Yes, you can, you are doing it!" I then remembered what Lynsey had told me. There is a stage in labour called the transition stage; it is where your body goes into a fight or flight mode, and it is yourself and the people around you that need to get you through this. But it is completely normal and natural to feel this. Remembering that this feeling was normal and that nothing was wrong and that I didn't need to panic but just stay focused, I pulled myself back together with the help of Shaune and our midwife. After 40 minutes of active pushing, our baby girl Penelope was delivered in the pool.

This is a memory I know will never fade. There was a brief moment before I reached into the water to bring Penelope out where she was looking up at me. I then reached in and pulled her towards my chest and looked over at Shaune, and we both just started to cry—our little girl Penelope was here at last.

I did it!!! We did it!

Within a few minutes of being sat at the edge of the pool, Penelope latched onto my nipple to be fed, and 20 minutes after she was born, my placenta detached itself in the water while I was still feeding Penelope. We couldn't have asked for a more perfect birth. Out of everything I had bought during my pregnancy in preparation, this was by far the best investment. Our birth was exactly what we chose and wanted, and I will eternally be grateful for this. I hope that one day we get to do it all again, as it is honestly the most surreal life-changing experience I have and will ever go through.

EDWIN

We always knew we wanted children and after a few years of marriage decided we would "try" to add to our family. We tried for a few months without success and then decided to give ourselves a break, went into a lockdown mid March 2020 and then found out I was pregnant on 5th April 2020, when I was trying to do a 5k Instagram trend and nearly passed out trying to beat 27 mins.

Due to lockdown there were no antenatal classes and hubby feeling pretty helpless started to google alternatives and came across hypnobirthing.
We found Lynsey online and contacted her and from our initial conversation to our last session it felt so comforting talking to someone in the know (who's also a mum and had practiced hypnobirthing herself).
Throughout the whole journey, I felt more relaxed but admittedly still didn't 100% believe mindset could play such a big part in a physical element of birth, that we had no experience in and couldn't practice.

What we loved was that the help and guidance wasn't just for mum but also dad on how to support as a birthing partner. The mp3s were amazing at relaxing us both at night, and the coping tips for when people gave unwelcome comments or advice were invaluable.

Although baby was 12 days late, I felt in control. I was offered induction on due date (without any need or reasoning), so with support and reassurance from Lynsey we declined. It was a decision we made together but I was ready for my body to do what it was meant to do (part of the course). The useful stories and facts from Lynsey put me in a really confident frame of mind. When I thought I was in labour, I checked Lynsey wasn't eating her dinner, and then shared things I never thought I'd share with someone I didn't know very well, and Lynsey was so supportive and a real tonic in such an uncertain time.

When the time came, I directed all midwives questions to Gary while I focused on my body. I got my water birth, and used my breathing techniques to really work through the knowledge that each surge was getting me one step closer to baby. I was in active labour for 45 mins and baby arrived happy and healthy. I still keep in touch with Lynsey now and baby is 2 soon. Had we known then what we know now, we would have spent double on what was, the best thing we've ever spent in parenthood. You spend money on the best rocking chairs and bouncers, for us, giving us the best chance of bringing our baby safely into the world was the best investment. If we ever had a second, I wouldn't hesitate to go on a refresher.

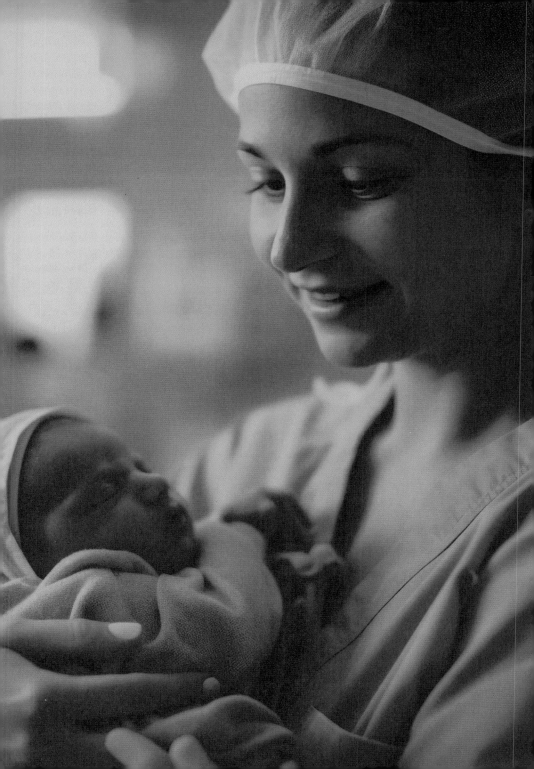

HOSPITAL BIRTH

The majority of births occur in NHS hospital maternity units, where midwives provide care, and doctors are available if needed. While retaining choices in your care, the hospital setting offers direct access to obstetricians and anesthetists for medical assistance, including epidurals. Neonatologists and a special care baby unit are on hand for any newborn issues.

Considerations

Before opting for a hospital birth, consider factors like potential postnatal ward placement, variation in midwife care, and a higher likelihood of interventions like epidurals, episiotomies, or forceps/ventouse deliveries.

Planning

Your midwife can assist in selecting the right hospital for you. Research each facility's offerings and choose based on your preferences. Be proactive in asking questions about maternity facilities, birth plans, pain relief options, equipment availability, birthing pools, and the hospital's policies.

Birth Questions to Ask:

Ask about maternity facility tours, discussing birth plans, pain relief options, available equipment, birthing pools, the presence of birthing partners, and the hospital's policy on induction, pain relief, and monitoring. Inquire about epidurals, post-birth arrangements, support for formula feeding, baby care, and visiting rules.

Flexibility:

Remember, you can change your birthing plan at any stage of pregnancy, ensuring your choice aligns with your evolving preferences.

KATIE

There were two lines on the stick – OMG, I'm pregnant! A thousand emotions surged through my mind at that moment. Standing and looking in the mirror, I realised I had the journey of a lifetime ahead, transitioning from the disbelief of becoming a mum to an immediate dash to Morrison's to buy another test. This marked just the beginning of the roller coaster ride we call motherhood.

Morning (or rather all-day sickness) quickly struck, persisting until the 24th week of my pregnancy, making me believe I would never eat again. Witnessing our baby on the screen during the first scan was a special moment, one I'll treasure forever. I felt the flutter everyone talks about, enjoyed watching my bump grow, but then fear started to creep in. I frantically Googled labour, avoiding Channel 4's "One Born Every Minute" – was it really going to be like that? Should I pack an extra-large box of throat sweets for the recovery? Not to worry, as I soon discovered "Born This Way" and met Lynsey, who initiated a completely new journey for me and our baby.

I cannot express how much of a worrywart I am; relaxation does not come naturally to me. Still, I was willing to try anything if it would help. Opening the door to Lynsey on a very wet Sunday afternoon, we instantly clicked. She was upbeat, passionate, and positive about birth. Over the next four weeks, we learned a lot about birth and how hypnobirthing could help prepare us. Two things stick out in my mind from our sessions:

Lynsey said a surge would last no longer than one minute.
If I don't relax and let my body naturally do it, I would be squashing my baby's head, as I wasn't listening to my body.
I remember watching birthing videos at the end of our sessions, seeing all the women look so relaxed. Honestly, I thought, "How can this work?" After every session, I wanted to believe it would work for me, but I doubted I could be that calm woman.

Lynsey talked about birth plans and being in control throughout. When it came to meeting my little girl, it wasn't like my birth plan. My waters unexpectedly broke 11 days before my due date, and 36 hours later, not even a twinge was felt. I didn't panic, as I felt in control due to hypnobirthing. We were called to the hospital to be induced, and somehow, I became one of those women on the videos we had watched. I listened to my body, naturally going into various positions. Even though it wasn't how I had written my birth plan, I felt in control. I focused on my waves, remembering Lynsey's comment: it's not going to be longer than two minutes. No pain relief was needed due to using my hypnobirthing techniques. Unfortunately, Katie was stuck towards the end, but I stayed calm and determined to meet my little bundle of joy. As Lynsey had advised, I asked to be talked through what would happen and still felt in control at the end. Finally, little Katie turned our world upside down at 8:02 am. I had done it! My baby was here!

I honestly can't describe labour, as everyone has a different birth story. Those who know me well understand how uptight, nervous, and panicky I can get. Still, during labour, I changed into a person I didn't even know; Hypnobirthing truly does prepare you. Lynsey was so positive and helpful, and I cannot thank her enough or recommend her more. She makes birthing exciting. Don't get me wrong; it's called labour for a reason, but preparation is key. In the months leading up to the birth, I was excited about labour as I felt Lynsey had given me all the correct techniques. I still feel the need to defend Hypnobirthing to many people – they say, "Oh, labour is awful, so painful." But as someone who panics about everything and wasn't 100% convinced how it would go until I was in labour, believe me, Hypnobirthing is the answer to a calm birthing experience. Thanks, Lynsey, for being a part of our journey.

BONNIE

I had a video call during the day with Mum, and once again, I was asked if I had felt any niggles, and I hadn't. We spoke about the membrane sweep that I was due to have on Friday (this was Monday), and Mum pointed out that every time I spoke about the sweep, I didn't seem happy. She was so right; it was really important to me that my baby came when they were ready, and when my body was ready too, even if I was desperate to meet them! I got off the phone and told Liam I had decided not to have the sweep; he was as supportive as always. Later that afternoon, I had the fleeting thought of 'I think I'm going to go today,' but I'd had that feeling before and nothing happened, so I didn't put too much stock in it.

We also tried out the TENS machine we had bought to help with the birth for the first time! It was a weird feeling - little did we know we'd be having a lot more of those over the next 48 hours! (Liam)

At about 10 pm, I thought I had my first surge; again, I just wasn't sure at all. I told Liam when he got into bed, and we just kind of thought, 'Oh well, let's see!'

We'd had a lovely dinner that night that Catherine (Jo's Step-mum) had prepared for us, so I thought we'd maybe just overeaten! (Liam)

By 1 am, I'd woken up briefly three times with a sort of minor cramp in my pelvis and lower back, and I thought... this must be the start of it! I felt the need to go to the loo, sat up, and my waters broke in bed. I made it to the bathroom, and I think I was a little shocked, so I kept walking back and forth until I realised I should let Liam know. I turned the bedroom light on and said, 'Bub, I think my waters have broken,' and it was like he rose from the dead comedy style; I've never seen him get up so fast!

I had only been asleep for an hour, but when I heard those words, I was wide awake as though I'd had a great night's sleep! (Liam)

We called the community midwife unit, and they said to come to the ward for a wee check - but told me that I'd probably get sent home again until my surges were closer together. We thought this might be the case anyway, and I had big plans - go for a walk, take a lovely bath and wash my hair (it really needed it haha!), eat some lovely food... we were tracking my surges with the Freya Surge app, and they were ranging from 3 - 7 minutes apart. We set up the TENS machine, and that definitely helped. Every time I had a surge, I rocked back and forth, using my hypnobirthing breathing techniques. By the time we got our stuff together to leave, it was about 2.15 am. We had opted for the RAH, which was a 20-minute drive for us, and I had four surges on the journey, and they were pretty sore - I think because I had to sit rather than move through the surge. I kept saying over and over in my head 'each surge only lasts a minute, and I could do anything for a minute'.

When we arrived at the RAH, Liam had to wait outside in the car, as I was only getting a checkup as far as the staff were concerned. I was asked to wait in a triage room until a midwife could see me. I was in that room on my own for about 20 minutes. I had popped my earphones in and was listening to Lynsey's audio recordings; they definitely helped me stay calm. I'd been listening to them regularly since Lynsey had given them to us and would speak along with them too. During this 20 minutes, my phone app started alerting me that I was in active labour! Again, I genuinely thought 'Nah, they'll check me over, and I'll go home, I'm going to wash my hair!'. Once the midwife took me through and had a look, the conversation went like:

"Right, is your partner here?"
"He's downstairs in the car; we're going home."
"Ok, let's call and get him up here."
"Oh! Should we bring our bags?"
"No, let's just get him up here."

What a huge difference in the 30 or so minutes between Jo leaving the car and me coming up to the room. From walking pretty much normally, she was now leaning over the bed, not a scrap on her bottom half, making noises I'd never heard before. Things were moving fast for sure! (Liam)

By about 3.30/4 am, I'd been wheeled through to the labour room - sitting in that wheelchair was the most uncomfortable thing! I do remember hitting the cool corridor on the way and asking if I could just stay there haha! By this time, my surges were very close together and very intense; I'd never felt anything like it. I chose to only have gas and air along with the hypnobirthing techniques we'd been taught (didn't get a chance to put pictures up haha!). Liam didn't let go of my hand the whole time; he was the most incredible support. Every time I felt like I couldn't do it anymore, I would look at him, and he would just know what to say or do. He would remind me to breathe; he'd tell me how well I was doing, how close I was to meeting our baby, he'd remind me of my affirmations; he was brilliant.

I genuinely had zero concept of time; I was only thinking as far as the wave I was having at the time. There were points where I was aware things weren't moving along, and I kept apologising to the midwives and Liam (haha!), and they kept telling me to shut up haha! The midwives were brilliant. Although I didn't get to go into the CMU due to staffing, I did have a CMU midwife, and the first thing she said to me was "you wanted an active labour, didn't you?". She was great, kept telling me when to move. I don't think I would have thought about it otherwise. Eventually, the midwives asked me to come off the gas and air; truth be told, I was losing steam/not pushing as hard right at the end of the surge, and my baby's head would go back the way. I looked at Liam and said, "I can't do this anymore," and he said, "that means they are almost here!" - my last four surges were done with nothing but a local anaesthetic downstairs as I had a small tear and an episiotomy to help get you out. Having a tear/episiotomy was one of my biggest fears about labour, but truthfully, I wasn't even aware of it happening at the time; I didn't feel it at all! The healing process afterward wasn't super wonderful, but it is now nothing but a distant memory.

Liam watched you arrive into the world at 7:20 am after four or so hours of active labour. I was too busy focusing everything I had on getting you out. It was absolutely the hardest and most empowering thing I've ever done, and I couldn't have done it without Liam, and we couldn't have done it without Lynsey's techniques!

As my daughter came out, Liam said, "it's a... girl?!" as he wasn't sure; the midwives confirmed he'd got it right. As she was placed into my arms, I looked at her, then Liam, and said, "Bonnie."

PHOEBE & FREYA

After getting married in 2019, we quickly fell pregnant with our first child. This was something we always wanted, and we excitedly discussed the parents we aspired to be and the future we envisioned. However, whenever a friend or relative had a baby, my initial questions were, "How sore was it?" or "Did you need stitches?" Amongst my close friends, it became apparent that I might be a bit apprehensive when it came to giving birth. Even after falling pregnant, I retained this nervous feeling about the birthing process and how I would endure this experience.

Upon attending my first midwife appointment, I expressed my nervousness about childbirth. My midwife recommended exploring hypnobirthing and joining a course. Following a discussion with Andrew, he mentioned a friend at work who had positive things to say about Hypnobirthing. At this point, we realised the need to invest in ourselves. Thus, our hypnobirthing journey with Lynsey began, and I can honestly say it significantly shaped our birthing experience. Fast forward two years, and we now have two amazing birth stories and two healthy, happy little girls.

The knowledge we gained through this experience was unparalleled. I learned to trust my body by understanding the why and what at each stage of my pregnancy. While it is beyond anyone's control to predict exactly what will happen during birth, I gained a new level of confidence in making informed decisions about my baby and my birth. With Lynsey's guidance, I felt prepared for whatever turn my birth might take.

Letting go of fears and progressively becoming more relaxed and calm in the lead-up to my births were crucial. For the main event, breathing techniques and a peaceful environment were my primary focus. The choices we made throughout our pregnancy and birth were a partnership decision. We extensively discussed our ideal birth scenario and what we would do if our birth took a different turn. Going into labour, I felt reassured, knowing that I had trust and confidence in Andrew to make decisions on behalf of our baby and me. Also, that he felt empowered to make these decisions as an equal partner.

I often describe Phoebe's birth as a long one. Initially, this might sound daunting, but people quickly learn that this lengthy process was completely controlled and managed through breathing techniques, resulting in nothing but a positive story. I woke up around 4 am on a Saturday morning with waves. Both of us were excited about the thought of our baby being born, but she was not ready. These waves gradually grew throughout the day. We went for a walk, returned home to watch Friends, and ate comfort food. After visiting our midwife-led unit, we discovered that our baby was not ready and returned home for the night. We stayed at home throughout the night and returned to the unit at 9 am. We had a pool room with dimmed lights, creating the perfect environment. We were fortunate to have a midwife who had trained in hypnobirthing and completely respected our choices. She asked questions like, "Would you prefer me to say waves or surges?" and "Do you want me to speak to you throughout each wave?" We remained in this room, with staff changing over three times throughout Sunday. Our final midwife was Caroline, a trainee midwife, who completely changed the atmosphere in the room. Her positive presence, guidance, and support gave me the motivation I needed in those final stages. In the end, I had my waters burst, and our first daughter quickly arrived into the world.

After having Phoebe, I couldn't wait to have more children. The feeling of achievement when birthing your baby is unforgettable. The sudden rush of love towards your child and your partner is something that cannot be explained. However, after falling pregnant again, I began to remember the length of time I birthed for, and fears quickly set in. Lynsey was able to teach me about the duration of each part of my labour and provide guidance on positions and movements that would help shorten and manage the labour time. During this pregnancy, I was informed that I was Strep B positive, which means there can be a chance of infection passed on during the birth between mother and baby. However, through hypnobirthing, I felt that I could question the options I was being given and remain calm when dealing with this.

Once again, around 4 am on a Saturday morning, pains started, and this time, instead of waking up with excitement at the thought of the arrival of my baby, I ignored them and went back to sleep. I woke up to nothing, so I walked down to our local park run. The waves started, and again, I ignored them while going back for tea and some cake with friends afterward. By lunchtime, the waves were more consistent, and I was able to gauge when I would need to make my way to the unit. When arriving at the unit, the door opened, and the midwife, Caroline, who delivered Phoebe, stood in front of me. I instantly felt safe. Having the same midwife again meant that she could pass on all my details from my first birth to the midwife that would look after us. Caroline knew we were highly passionate about hypnobirthing and when I began to show a bit of doubt about my birth and the pain, she corrected me. She said, "You can do this and you will do this. No more negative talk." I felt blessed to have her support to reinforce what we had learned with Lynsey. Caroline sorted me out with my antibiotics for my Strep B, and I was placed into a birthing room. This room was the perfect setup. We were now in full control of our birth. As a team, we breathed together, got comfortable, and when I knew it was time, I got into the pool. I experienced the transition period and knew that our baby was going to arrive soon. As the midwives looked over, I birthed my baby. She floated to the top of the pool, and we put our arms around her. I did it!

We practiced the same techniques during our second pregnancy, and I cannot stress how important this was. To be able to refresh our skills, reflect on our first experience, and prepare for our second pregnancy played a huge part in another positive birth story. The constant reinforcement of the skills learned throughout the hypnobirthing experience makes the end result a success. I believe that the pregnancy journey and the preparation are equally important to the birth, making for a positive birthing experience.

ARABELLA

I want to begin by expressing that birthing your child is one of the most natural things a human mother can do. Our bodies are designed to nurture, nourish, and support our little ones before their journey into the world.

The reason I'm sharing this is to reassure you that your body knows what it's doing; it will support you. Regardless of whether you're four weeks into your pregnancy or 40 weeks, trust that you've got this.

My pregnancy was a happy surprise. Initially, in 2017, I had been told that I was infertile and wouldn't be able to conceive naturally due to my polycystic ovary syndrome. My ovaries were full of cysts, and I hadn't been having periods. However, I also know the human body is capable of incredible healing.

In 2019, my fiancé and I decided to start trying for a family in the spring of 2020. I changed my diet and lifestyle to correct the PCOS hormonal imbalances and create as fertile a body as I could.

Then the happy accident happened! We fell pregnant in January 2020 before we'd even properly started trying.

I thought I'd have a lot longer before our wee one would be due, so I hadn't read up on everything I would have wanted to on pregnancy, the journey ahead, or birth. But I did know of a few experts in their field who do incredible work with expectant mothers, so I chose to work with them during my pregnancy.

One was my herbalist, and the other is the incredible Lynsey, a

Hypnobirthing midwife and Doula.

As a first-time Mum, I was nervous about what was ahead but also trusted that everything would be okay because that's what I believe; everything will always work out.

Lynsey is such a welcoming, caring, and genuinely delightful human to be around. She instantly puts you at ease and has such a passion for her work that you can't help but be excited in her presence.

I didn't actually realise how thorough her hypnobirthing course would be, and for both my fiancé and me, it hugely put us at ease for the journey ahead. Equipped with all the knowledge and practical skills from Lynsey, I felt confident about giving birth, my choices within the hospital, and any options if a plan B was needed. It was also a lot of fun learning about the whole process, the amazing anatomy of the female reproductive system, and the specifics of what went on during the birth process.

So I'm not going to sugarcoat my birth journey...for me, it was long, intense, and exhausting. I had what's called a stop-start labour when your contractions start and then stop to then start again. Wednesday night about 10 pm the week before my daughter was due, the contractions kicked in. Using the techniques I'd learned, I was able to make myself more comfortable and managed to get a couple of hours of sleep in the early hours of Thursday only to wake to no more contractions. That evening around 10 pm again, the next wave came and kept me up overnight until Friday when I managed about an hour's sleep.

Being able to have breathing and relaxation skills specific to my body's needs kept me going on such little sleep. By Friday dinnertime, I felt exhausted, very emotional but still knowing that it was all going to be okay. Labour properly started about 11 pm Friday.

Throughout that night, I moved between the couch, my birthing ball, and the floor. As the contractions came more quickly, rather than feeling nervous, I actually felt excited. By 9 am, I woke my partner, and it was time to drop our pets off at the in-laws and go to the hospital.

We got to my in-laws just before 11, and the contractions had slowed down but felt more intense. By this point, I was feeling very emotional from the lack of sleep. I remembered Lynsey had said to stay hydrated and fed, so my wonderful man was on hand to help me. The day seemed to go on forever as the contractions slowed increased. Come 10 pm, and I was a bit of an emotional wreck.

Low on calories, aching from no sleep and the physical work of my body preparing for birth, I made my fiancé drive us to the hospital. When the midwife checked, I was only 2 cm dilated.

I felt sore, I just wanted to have my baby, but I also had no interest in any interventions. So when I was offered a "wee sweep," I continued my hypnobirthing breathing work and confidently said no. Whether you have a quick and easy labour or a long drawn-out one, being able to stay in a clear state of mind to make the right choices for you is hugely empowering, and I would not have been able to do that without Lynsey's help and support.

Back at my in-laws, I continued to contract into the early hours. One thing I haven't mentioned is my pain threshold is pretty low; I didn't even like getting my eyebrows waxed! So by the time my contractions were 7 minutes apart, I'd had enough. Straight back to the hospital and into a wheelchair to get me to maternity assessment.

The actual ward was full and had no spare beds yet, but according to the midwife, I probably had 5 hours to go. My baby had other plans.

While up on the bed with just gas and air, I said we still wanted the water birth room and was told we could go there in a few hours when I was further dilated.

After less than an hour of being on the bed, I went into transition. Ladies, for me, this was REALLY intense! It lasted just moments while I screamed, then was told by the midwife to take it easy on the gas and air.

Inside my head, I cussed her every name under the sun because you know your own body, and trust me, when your baby is coming, you know! She told me it was still a few more hours.

I continued to breathe through the whole process, and the next thing, just 20 minutes later, I felt my baby coming down the birth canal as my legs involuntarily came up to my chest. The next second, my fiancé's face reappeared from looking under the covers and said there's a head!

As my daughter quickly made her way into the world, my partner grabbed the midwives who came rushing in to finish the delivery.

My body was intact albeit sore, and I was given this perfect, squishy little human. My baby girl.

There had been no interventions, no difficulties, and no big stress. I felt absolutely spent but I was holding my perfect little bundle along with my wonderful man.

Giving birth naturally was what I wanted. We didn't make it to the birthing pool or even the maternity ward, but my little one made her way into the world as nature intended.

Trusting in my body and having the tools to make the experience one of discomfort rather than suffering was so empowering. Having a natural birth is not going to be without pain, but using the breathing work, visualization, and techniques that Lynsey teaches will support you mentally, physically, and emotionally through your journey.

You'll be in a place to make confident informed decisions, as well as knowing what to expect.

From Gary, Arabella, and me, thank you so much for not only being a huge part of our journey but for allowing us to have what we needed to experience such a wonderful birth.

And to you, the reader, you've absolutely got this. Enjoy your journey, prepare for everything, and trust in yourself and your incredible body.

SAM

We chose to participate in the Born This Way Hypnobirthing classes with Lynsey upon discovering that we were expecting our third child. Both my partner and I carried some lingering anxiety about the birth, stemming from the fairly traumatic experience we had four years earlier when our wonderful twin daughters were born. Initially, we hadn't fully grasped the extent of the trauma from that experience. However, early in the Hypnobirthing classes, we gained a comprehensive understanding of our previous birth and recognised where things had gone wrong, leading to the erosion of our control over the situation.

The tools, techniques, and advice provided throughout the course proved to be invaluable during the birth of our son, Sam. In stark contrast to the birth of the twins, this experience was truly magical. Even though we found ourselves executing plan C or D from our birth plan, it never felt like we had lost control of the situation. I have never felt so calm in such a position, and we owe this remarkable sense of calmness to Lynsey at Born This Way. Thanks to her guidance, we now have a wonderfully positive birth story to share, a stark contrast to our initial birthing experience.

KIARA

Throughout the challenging year of 2020, where uncertainties abounded for everyone, the prospect of becoming first-time parents loomed as the most significant concern for Liam and me. Although it was our dream, anxiety was a constant companion. Despite having read numerous books and equipped ourselves with all the necessary gadgets, the prospect of giving birth left us feeling inadequately prepared.

Lynsey emerged as a beacon of reassurance, alleviating many of our fears. We consider ourselves incredibly fortunate to have discovered Lynsey and her Born This Way Hypnobirthing programme, which, in my opinion, transformed my entire perspective not only on birth but also on everyday life. I continue to embrace a positive mindset regularly, wearing my "positive pants" and using mindfulness for self-regulation. The program, designed for childbirth, supported me in more ways than I could have imagined, especially during such tumultuous times.

Both Liam and I initially harboured anxiety about the birthing process, viewing it as something to endure, and then we'd get to enjoy the joy of having a baby. I never thought I could perceive birth as an exciting, empowering process. Words like 'scary' and 'painful' initially came to mind. However, by the last session, I felt excitement, positivity, and anticipation for the process.

With Lynsey's guidance, we delved into mindfulness sessions, explored various birth options, crafted our birth plan collaboratively, and posed an abundance of questions. I eagerly anticipated our calming, peaceful sessions, and it was the only antenatal program where I saw Liam fully engaged (after dosing through others!). The Born This Way sessions are active, engaging, and involve you as part of the process. Trust in it, and it will work.

Feeling immensely empowered, I navigated through many hours of initial contractions without pain relief, using my 'Place of Peace' as a focal tool. Confidence in my choices allowed me to select the options I deemed best for both the baby and myself, ensuring the safe and, at times, calm arrival of our beautiful baby girl.
We have conveyed our gratitude to Lynsey and are truly indebted to her support and program. Should we be blessed with another baby one day, we would be immensely grateful to refresh our knowledge with Lynsey when the time comes.

TOM

When I discovered I was pregnant with my second child, the initial joy was overshadowed by the haunting memory of a traumatic birth experience with my son three years earlier. The mere discussion of childbirth would trigger panic within me, often reducing me to tears at the mere thought. The idea of pleading for a planned c-section seemed like the only viable option. At the recommendation of a friend, I reluctantly explored hypnobirthing, a concept I was unfamiliar with and initially sceptical of. Desperation drove me to try anything that could alleviate my fears. Little did I know that learning about hypnobirthing would turn out to be one of the best decisions I've ever made.

Within just a couple of sessions, my confidence soared, and a newfound sense of relaxation allowed me to embrace my pregnancy with minimal fear. While that alone would have sufficed, by the time my due date arrived, I was genuinely excited about going into labour—a sentiment unimaginable six months earlier.

On the day I went into labour, I felt well-prepared. After a brief stint at home, I sensed it was time to head to the hospital. Upon arrival, they informed me that I was already 5cm dilated, ready to transition to the labour ward. Entering the birthing pool immediately, I remained there until after delivering my baby. While it wasn't exactly pain-free, I experienced not a single ounce of fear. I maintained composure and confidence, trusting that my body knew precisely what to do. Employing relaxation and breathing techniques, along with intermittent use of gas and air, I coped well with the pain. My husband and midwife, seemingly unoccupied, witnessed me quietly navigating through the process in the pool. Other staff members entering the room would remark on the remarkable calmness.

After five hours in the water, my beautiful 9lb 4oz baby boy entered the world, and I vividly recall the surge of oxytocin—a true love bubble. I distinctly remember thinking that, if asked to give birth again the very next day, I absolutely could. On that day, I felt an unprecedented strength and empowerment, marking a pinnacle in my life.

MIRREN

The prospect of giving birth always filled me with terror. When I discovered I was pregnant, it triggered a mix of emotions—excitement intertwined with sheer dread at the thought of bringing this baby into the world. Initially, I harboured the notion of opting for a c-section, considering it the easier route—an indication of my lack of knowledge at the time.

We decided to attend group sessions with Lynsey, recommended by a work colleague, and it proved to be a transformative experience. My perspective on childbirth underwent a complete overhaul. Delving into the stages of labour and acquiring various tips and tricks not only made the process less daunting but also empowered me to make informed decisions. The relaxation techniques introduced during the sessions became a valuable resource, particularly towards the end of my pregnancy. Astonishingly, my preference shifted from desiring a c-section to aspiring for a water birth.

The actual birth unfolded rapidly, with my waters breaking and the baby arriving within a mere 4 hours. Upon reaching the hospital, I discovered I was fully dilated, albeit missing out on the water birth I had hoped for. Despite this, I felt well-informed and conscious of the unfolding events. Utilising the relaxation techniques during the journey to the hospital helped me maintain composure.

Reflecting on my birthing experience, I can confidently say it was an overall positive journey, and much of that credit goes to hypnobirthing and Lynsey's invaluable guidance. I wholeheartedly recommend Lynsey to anyone grappling with concerns about labour and childbirth. Her sessions instill peace of mind in the lead-up to the big day—a priceless gift in my eyes!

GLORIA

I found the idea of giving birth quite terrifying, likely influenced by watching numerous episodes of One Born Every Minute. The prospect of my baby being delivered through natural means filled me with fear. However, my perception underwent a significant transformation after my first session with Lynsey. The relaxation tracks provided during the pregnancy became a source of comfort, not only aiding relaxation but also instilling excitement for the impending day. No longer did fear dominate; I was prepared and ready for the challenge, eagerly anticipating the experience.

My labour spanned 37 hours, initially aiming for a home birth. However, the course had prepared me to navigate obstacles, emphasising the importance of understanding and deciding on the right birth for the day, rather than blindly adhering to a predetermined plan. After 12 intense hours at home, I opted to transfer to the hospital.

During the first 12 hours of labour, I employed a combination of gas and air, a tens machine, deep breathing, and tingle-touch massages from my partner, Scott. Remaining active and trusting my instincts, I moved through various positions. Despite experiencing established labour, I wasn't dilating, prompting a decision to induce at the hospital after initially declining the intervention.

Having some diamorphine at the hospital helped me rest between surges. The subsequent 25 hours involved using hypnobirthing techniques, with Scott's support as an empowered birth partner. A carefully curated playlist lost its relevance to the effectiveness of hypnobirthing tracks in helping me zone out and endure the hospital setting.

When the urge to push arose, I felt determined. Despite the midwives suggesting intervention, I insisted on birthing without assistance. The pushing phase, initially feared, concluded rapidly, with Gloria Mae Johnston arriving without intervention, bringing an overwhelming rush of endorphins.

While hypnobirthing drastically altered my perception of labour, making it a positive challenge, my husband also attests to its transformative impact. I recommend hypnobirthing to every expectant mother, a sentiment echoed by my husband. The course not only changed my approach to labour but also empowered me to question medical professionals when making informed choices, as exemplified during the breech baby scenario at 40+2 weeks. The hypnobirthing techniques equipped me to remain calm during a procedure, avoiding unnecessary interventions and impressing the medical team with my composure. The course, delivered by Born This Way Hypnobirthing, has been an invaluable and transformative experience.

FIONN

In mid-January 2022, my partner, Fergus, and I discovered that our family would be expanding with the anticipated arrival of tiny toes in September. Initially, we were overjoyed, but as the due date approached, the realization set in that we were unprepared for the imminent birth of our baby. Lacking practical knowledge beyond television dramatizations and conversations with family and friends, both Fergus and I felt a sense of uncertainty about what to expect during this significant life event.

Upon expressing my concerns to a friend, Lynsey was recommended for her excellent knowledge and support during pregnancy. Intrigued by the positive experience my friend had, I eagerly contacted Lynsey for more information. Following discussions, my partner and I enrolled in a four-week, in-person group course when I was approximately 25 weeks pregnant. Before the first session, I was optimistic and excited, while Fergus, being unsure of what to expect, was more apprehensive.

Over the course of ten hours spanning four weeks, Lynsey provided us with invaluable information, leaving both Fergus and me feeling well-informed and confident about the upcoming birth. One of the key lessons we learned was that we were in control of our own birthing experience, possessing choices we had not previously realised. This newfound sense of empowerment allowed us to discuss our preferences before the birth, enabling us to be realistic about potential interventions if necessary. Feeling safe with Fergus aware of and supportive of my wishes, I gained a deeper understanding of the importance of making our birthing experience positive, regardless of its progression.

Hypnobirthing, initially sought to alleviate my nerves, provided Fergus with considerable knowledge as well. Through sessions, he grasped the purposeful and significant role he would play as my birthing partner. The practices of partner massage and listening to positive affirmations, as recommended by Lynsey, became integral to our preparations. Fergus, overseeing the birthing plan and setting up the labour room, contributed to a calm atmosphere towards the end of my pregnancy and throughout our birthing journey.

Around 9 pm on September 11th, 2022, Fergus and I headed to the Princess Royal Hospital as I wasn't feeling well, experiencing reduced foetal movement and a rising temperature. Unaware that I was in labour, the unexpected revelation that I had Covid-19 heightened our concern for our baby's safety. Employing deep breathing to stay calm, further examination revealed I was indeed in labour. Dilation progressed more than expected, prompting an immediate transfer to a labour room.

Within the room, I confidently voiced my preferences, from requesting a birthing ball and dimmed lights to creating a comfortable atmosphere. Fergus handed over the birthing plan, crafted with Lynsey's template, outlining the most important aspects for both of us. Utilising the "Born This Way Meditation Track," I maintained deep breathing on the birthing ball, aiming for mobility within the room. Fergus supported me with a gentle partner massage during moments of respite, allowing me to endure the intense waves comfortably.
As the waves intensified, I requested gas and air, adhering to my birth plan's preference for medication that wouldn't cross the placenta unless absolutely essential. However, as our third stage of labour progressed, our baby's heart rate dropped, leading to a discussion with the doctor. Following a conversation with Fergus, I consented to an episiotomy to facilitate a safe birth. At 4.25 am on September 12th, our beautiful baby boy, Fionn John-James MacGregor, was born.

Throughout the labour, I heeded Lynsey's advice, listening to my body and allowing the natural progression of our baby down the birth canal. Despite the fatigue, I consented to the injection for placenta birth, choosing the option best suited for me at the time. Fionn's skin-to-skin contact directly after birth was a magical experience in a safe, calm, and positive environment.

Fergus and I are profoundly grateful to Lynsey for empowering us during this momentous life event. The birth of our incredible baby boy was filled with joyous memories, everything we had wished for and more. We wholeheartedly recommend Lynsey to expecting friends, recognising her impact on our lives in a wonderful way. Thank you, Lynsey, for your lasting influence on our journey.

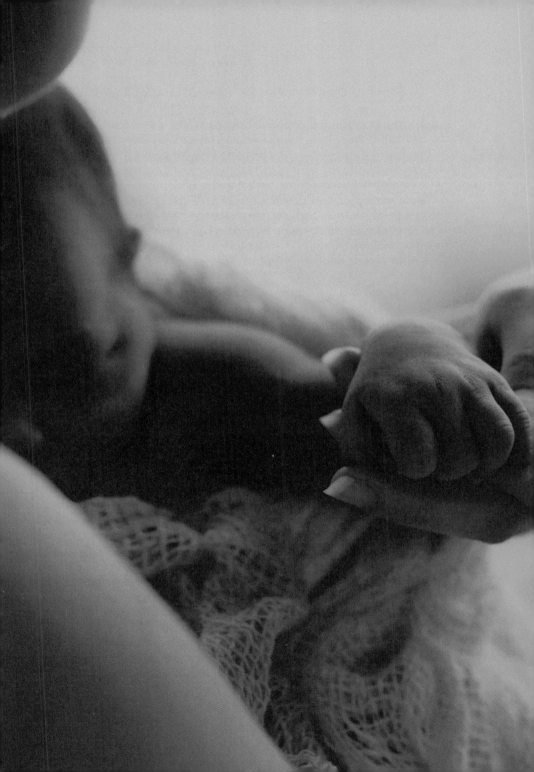

ASSISTED BIRTH

Assisted birth is when forceps or ventouse are used in the last stage of birth to help the baby to be born.

Assisted birth may be recommended when:

- You feel exhausted
- If your baby in not in the optimum position to birth as assistance can help the baby to turn.
- If you have an epidural on board and can't feel the sensation to push baby down the birth canal.
- If there are concerns for either you or baby's wellbeing in the final stage of labour.

Both instruments, forceps and ventouse, are employed only when appropriate pain relief is administered. If a woman has an epidural during labour, she would be numb, unable to feel anything. Without an epidural, local or spinal anaesthetic is given to numb the vaginal and vulval area.

For a ventouse or forceps-assisted birth, the woman is positioned on her back with legs in stirrups. The bed's bottom is removed, allowing the care provider to perform the procedure closely. A catheter is inserted to reduce the need for bathroom trips under anaesthetic.

Forceps, resembling curved, smooth salad tongs, are placed on each side of the baby's head and connected at a handle. The doctor guides the baby out as the mother pushes.

Ventouse, a suction cup, is applied to the baby's head, creating a seal, and the doctor guides the baby out while the mother pushes simultaneously. Ventouse isn't recommended for babies under 34 weeks gestation due to their softer heads, which may lead to bruising or injury.

In some births it may be required to perform an episiotomy (a cut in the perineum skin under local anaesthetic) this is to make space to get the instruments in place.

Assisted birth can seem a daunting prospect for many in pregnancy. As with so many things about birth, assisted birth stories are rarely positive ones and I want to show you that isn't always the case.
We are so lucky to have skilled doctors that are trained in performing

assisted births as their skills can save lives.

There are some things that can help reduce the chance of requiring an instrumental birth.

These include:

- Being in positions where you are upright, forward and open. This increases the space baby has by up to 30% and helps gravity assist baby down the birth canal.
- If you are having a low risk healthy pregnancy (sometimes referred to a green pathway) consider giving birth in a birthing centre or home birth setting as there is less chance of interventions including ventouse and forceps.
- Avoid having an epidural as your form of pain relief. Epidural anaesthesia means your mobility and freedom to move about in labour is restricted, this can hinder the baby moving down the birth canal. If you do choose to have an epidural a top tip is to wait for a while after you are fully dilated before you begin to push as the extra time will help baby's head descend down the birth canal.
- Having a continuous support partner in labour helps you feel safe and helps your birth hormones release more effectively. This can be your partner but evidence shows having a birth doula (a non-medical birth professional who offers continuous emotional and physical support for you and your birth partner) can reduce the need for assisted birth.

Assisted birth is not something that can just happen it can only be done with informed consent. If this type of birth is recommended remember to use your B.R.A.I.N. Acronym to help with your decision making.

Make sure to ask:

- Why an instrumental birth is recommended?
- Which instrument is preferred in your case and why?
- Is there any risks to you or your baby?
- Is there an alternative option that may be better?

SOPHIA

Nine days before my due date, I began experiencing subtle "tightenings" occurring approximately every 40 to 50 minutes. Sensing the onset of something significant, I prepared for the day, heading out for lunch with a friend to stimulate my oxytocin. Upon returning home, I spent quality time with my partner, dog, and both our families. Later that night, during a shower, I attended to my hair and applied tan, before retiring to bed to watch Love Island, intending to enhance the flow of oxytocin. Around 10-11 pm, my contractions increased in frequency, disrupting my ability to sleep through them. Employing my tens machine and bouncing on an exercise ball, I managed to catch 3-4 hours of sleep. At 6 am, I contacted the hospital, expressing my belief that I was in labour. Despite having dealt with high blood pressure during my pregnancy, which was currently stable, I opted to stay at home, a decision the hospital agreed with for the time being.

Throughout the day, I laboured at home, using my tens machine and employing hypnobirthing breathing techniques as my contractions ranged from 3 to 12 minutes apart. Between contractions, I engaged in various activities, including watching films, conversing with visiting family, enjoying good food, soaking up the sun, and playing with my dog. By around 10 pm, feeling the need to go to the hospital, my partner and I shared light-hearted banter during the journey, with him playfully navigating speed bumps, claiming to assist in moving the baby.

Upon reaching the hospital, a midwife checked my cervix and found me to be 4 cm dilated, expressing surprise at my calm demeanor attributed to hypnobirthing breathing. Due to my high blood pressure, the midwife recommended going to the labour ward, breaking my waters, and I agreed.

I arrived at the labour ward around 1:30 am and was offered pain relief options. Opting for an epidural and gas and air, I had planned the epidural in advance to help manage my blood pressure. The midwife broke my waters and monitored the baby until the anaesthetist administered the epidural around 3 am, after a brief delay due to an emergency c-section. Despite the delay, I continued using breathing techniques, gas and air, and the tens machine. My attitude towards labour, once terrifying, had transformed, and I found myself genuinely enjoying the experience.

At 4:40 am, the epidural was administered, allowing me to rest before the anticipated arrival of my baby. At 6:30 am, the midwife informed me that my daughter was showing signs of distress, and as I was only 6 cm dilated, suggested a c-section. Requesting alternatives, a fetal blood sample was proposed, with results indicating it was safe to proceed with a vaginal birth. By 8 am, I was fully dilated and ready to push.

However, another fetal blood sample was taken, revealing concerns, prompting a discussion with my midwife about safe delivery options. Despite initially opting for forceps, I later agreed to the safest option for my daughter, a c-section. The doctor arrived, and my daughter was born in just two pushes, surprising me with the speed and ensuring her safe arrival.

I expressed deep gratitude to Lynsey for imparting knowledge and relaxation techniques, transforming my initial fear of labour into a positive experience. On the same day as my daughter's birth, I declared my love for the process and expressed willingness to go through it again. This newfound perspective was attributed to the breathing techniques that guided me through each contraction, knowing that every wave brought us closer to meeting our baby girl.

CAMILLE

When we found out we were pregnant, we were so excited! As the pregnancy progressed, I started thinking more and more about labour and birth and realised how daunting the whole process seemed and actually how little I knew about it! I was so scared about the pain and the traumatic stories I had heard that I'd convinced myself my birth story would be the same. Even the thought of going into labour made my stomach go into knots, and it felt so overwhelming!

I didn't want my experience to be like this, and Lynsey was recommended to me by friends, so I got in touch! The hypnobirthing course was invaluable to myself and my husband, and I fully believe it's what got me through my birthing experience. Lynsey taught me the mechanics of birth—something I had never even heard about. Knowing how birth worked and what my body was doing made the process seem so much less daunting. The relaxation techniques I used through pregnancy and beyond helped me manage my anxiety throughout. After the course with Lynsey, I started to feel excited about the birth of my baby and knew the end goal was to meet our little girl! I'd say the most valuable part for us was the confidence Lynsey gave us to make decisions for ourselves and that it was okay to take time to make important decisions about birth and what would work for us.

I was induced at 38 weeks due to reduced movements. I used the BRAIN acronym to come to the decision that induction was going to be the best decision for us and our baby after weighing up all the options. Throughout my induction process, which was longer than expected, I was able to remain relaxed and calm using Lynsey's techniques. If I felt unsure about something, I had the confidence to ask one of the midwives and make informed decisions about my labour.

As we know, not all things in life go to plan, and my labour did end in an episiotomy and ventouse delivery, which wasn't in my initial plans! However, throughout the full process, I felt calm and confident, and I look back at my labour with such happy memories, so much so I'm ready to do it again, after a refresher course obviously!

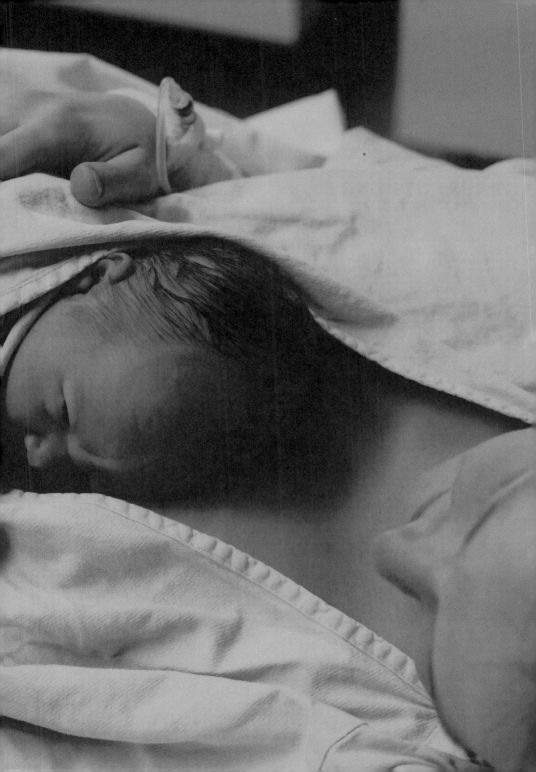

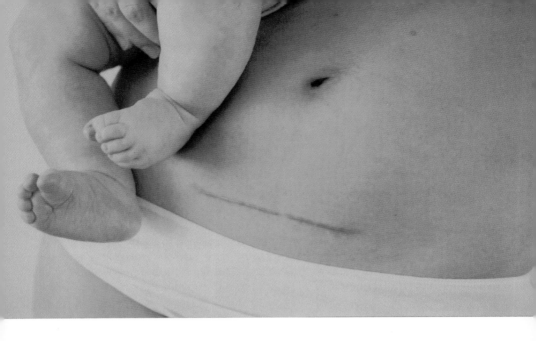

VBAC

VBAC, or Vaginal Birth After Cesarean, is an option for women who have had a previous cesarean section and wish to give birth vaginally with a subsequent pregnancy.

It's important to note that VBAC feasibility depends on various factors, such as the reason for the previous cesarean, the type of incision made, and overall maternal health.

Benefits of VBAC:

1. **Reduced Risks:** VBAC is associated with lower risks of infection, blood loss, and complications compared to repeat cesarean sections.
2. **Shorter Recovery:** Recovery time after a vaginal birth is generally shorter than after a cesarean section, allowing mothers to resume regular activities more quickly.
3. **Lower Risk for Future Pregnancies:** Successful VBAC may reduce the likelihood of complications in future pregnancies.

Considerations and Challenges:

1. **Risk Assessment:** Healthcare providers carefully assess the risk factors involved, considering the reason for the previous cesarean and the type of uterine incision.
2. **Monitoring During Labour:** Monitoring the babies heartbeat is recommended to promptly identify any signs of uterine rupture, although this is a very rare occurrence. This affects around one in 200 women trying for a VBAC. That risk is increased two to three fold if labour is induced.
3. **Hospital Policies:** Some hospitals have specific policies or guidelines regarding VBAC, so it's crucial to discuss these with your healthcare provider.
4. **Emergency Preparedness:** Emergency resources, including an operating room and medical staff capable of performing a cesarean section, should be readily available during a VBAC attempt.

Decision-Making:

Expectant mothers should engage in open communication with their healthcare providers to discuss the feasibility of VBAC based on individual circumstances. Factors such as maternal preferences, medical history, and the provider's experience play a role in making an informed decision.

Ultimately, VBAC is a viable option for many women, but the decision should be personalised, taking into account both the potential benefits and risks.

LYLE

My birth experience with my first son was something I took a little time to come to terms with as it was everything I didn't want to go through. I was due on December 19th, 2018, and I focused so much on the date as it was going to be close to Christmas day. I got to 9 days overdue and received a call from the hospital to be induced at 11 pm at night. At the time, I didn't know my options, so I jumped at the chance to get things going to finally meet our baby!! I had no idea how things would happen or what to expect, and after a long labour, our baby's heart rate was dipping too low and too often that it was advised an emergency section would be safest, and that is how our beautiful healthy baby boy Harry was born on December 29th, 2018. It took me time to come to terms with the fact that I never got the "Natural" birth or felt positive about my experience. However, I had this beautiful healthy baby boy to shower love over, so I soon put those thoughts out of my mind, but I knew if I was to go on and have more children that I would love a different experience.

I started following Born this way Hypnobirthing on Instagram way before I was even thinking about a second baby. I saw Lynsey's page via a friend's recommendation and followed her page. When I fell pregnant at the end of 2021, I knew I wanted to book in with Lynsey to do her course even though I was in Aberdeen, and I knew it probably wouldn't be in person, so I booked in straight away.

After the first class via zoom, I instantly knew I was going to love both Lynsey and the content; everything felt right! All the material just made sense. Throughout the classes which my husband, Greig, also attended, we learned how my body would prepare for birth, the stages it would go through, and how it was more than capable of birthing my baby even after my first being a section. We both loved the relaxation and learning the tingle touch massages, and I especially loved the breathing techniques which I managed to practice a lot when I failed to dodge Lego toys left on our floor!! They really helped me calm myself and breathe through any discomfort, along with the pressure points techniques; those skills were invaluable to me during my birth.

My due date came and went, but at no point did I focus on a date. I kept calm, relaxed and used the techniques from the handbook and affirmations to remind myself that my baby will come when they are ready and I was more than capable of birthing the baby I had lovingly carried and grew all these months. I was offered my first sweep at 40 + 1; however, I politely refused as I was in no rush and didn't feel that I needed to intervene any time soon; my midwife was massively supportive of my choices and respected all the decisions I was making. Days came and went, but I continued to listen to my relaxation and affirmation tracks and enjoyed long soaks in the bath with essential oils. I had made the decision that I would let myself get to 42 weeks and if nothing had happened by then, I would look into informed induction options.

I accepted the option of a sweep at 40 + 3 then another at 40 + 8; however, nothing was instant, but I was OK with this. I had a growth scan to make sure all was well, and it was, so I was happy to wait it out and give my baby and body a chance.

The morning of June 10th came, and at 05:40 am, I started feeling some tightenings which were very regular and growing in intensity over the morning. I was reluctant to make any calls as I was a little scared of jinxing anything, but by 9 am, my waves were stronger and frequent, and I had passed a lot of mucus, so I knew something was happening. My in-laws came and picked up our older son, and we made a phone call to the midwife team as I had opted for a home birth and wanted to go forward with that choice. The midwife came out to us at 13:30 and examined me; I was reluctant to have anyone come sooner in case I was told I wasn't far along or dilated far and that would play on my mind and put me back mentally so I waited as long as I could. When the midwife came out I was told I was 4-5 cms so decided to get in the pool and use some gas and air. Up until that point I used a comb to squeeze into my palm which I learned through Lynsey, and it was very effective; I switched to the TENS machine which I also found really worked for me and then eventually got into the water.

I found it invaluable that Greig had done the hypnobirthing course alongside me as he knew exactly what to look and watch for and knew when I needed something without me even asking. As a wave was approaching all I needed was one hand on Greig to take me to a place of peace and get me through. The techniques I had learned through the born this way course got me through every single wave that came and went and I trusted that my body could get through anything and birth my baby. I rested in between waves and was in such a state of relaxation that I wasn't really aware of what was happening around me. I used a diffuser to fill the room with my chosen scent (clary sage) and played my tracks in between songs I had chosen on a playlist. By 18:32 our baby was born in the pool behind my sofa in our living room. I lifted my baby through my legs (I birthed on my knees) and held another beautiful baby boy on my chest, Lyle. I couldn't quite believe that it was all done and I had done it exactly how I had planned and hoped. By 21:45 I was all sorted, showered and feeding our new baby boy in my bed with a cup of tea. I was feeling so empowered and on cloud 9, even like I could do it all again!

I honestly don't think I would have had the birth I did without the Born this way hypnobirthing course; it was invaluable to my husband and me. The knowledge we gained about birth ensured we could make the most informed decisions for us and gave me the most important skills to help me through my labour. If I ever do it all again, I would want to do it the exact same way. I look back on my second son's birth with fond memories, and I love thinking and talking about it. It was such a positive experience, and I am so grateful for the knowledge and skills I gained which I still use in my everyday life.

SOFIA MAY

We were so thrilled about our second pregnancy, excitement filled our hearts, especially considering the joy our son had brought into our lives.

Opting for a VBAC (vaginal birth after cesarean) this time, I, being considered "high risk" due to a previous section, received exceptional support from my consultant. Determined and focused, my ideal birth vision became a powerful motivation.

The Hypnobirthing homework involved scripting our ideal birth, a moving experience that made the impending reality feel more tangible. Labour commenced on August 26th, accompanied by occasional niggles that evolved into waves. Despite being past my due date, I refrained from fixating on numbers and switched my focus to being as relaxed as possible.

As waves intensified, my husband timed them while we created a serene ambiance with candles and my birthing playlist. Surprisingly calm, I assumed these waves would settle, allowing me to sleep soon.

Upon contacting the midwife-led unit and observing the frequency of waves, we embarked on the journey to the hospital, during which I maintained focus with my hypnobirthing breathing techniques. Even a pit stop at McDonald's for a coffee for my husband didn't disrupt the serene atmosphere.

At the hospital, we met Margaret, a hypnobirthing midwife, whose calming presence eased the transition. After being examined and observed, Margaret offered acupuncture and allowed me to continue in the lounge. Focused on my breathing and massage from my husband, I entered the dreamlike experience of transitioning to the pool.

As the intensity increased, I reached the transition stage, feeling an intense pressure as my membranes ruptured. Focused on the song 'A Thousand Years' by Christina Perri, I moved through the final stages, and before I knew it, our beautiful girl was safely in my arms.

With no drugs, just breathing techniques, a supportive husband, and an amazing midwife, the perfect birth unfolded. Our family feels complete, and I'm grateful for the right birth on that remarkable day.

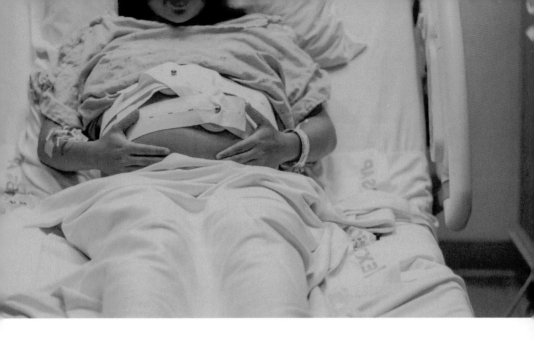

INDUCTION

Induction of labour is a medical procedure conducted to initiate or stimulate contractions of the uterus, bringing about the onset of labour. This intervention is typically recommended when the health of the mother or baby is at risk, or when the pregnancy has surpassed the estimated due date.

In the UK, NICE guidelines advise induction of labour at 41 weeks. When proposing induction, it is crucial to acknowledge that women can choose to proceed with, delay, decline, or halt an induction. Respecting the woman's decision, even if healthcare professionals disagree, is paramount, and personal views should not influence the care provided.

Here is a comprehensive overview of the induction of labour process:

- **Assessment:** Before deciding on induction, the healthcare provider assesses the overall health of the mother and the baby. This involves a physical examination, a review of medical history, and monitoring the baby's heartbeat. A vaginal examination is also performed to assess the cervix and determine its readiness for induction.

- **Cervical Ripening:** If the cervix is not sufficiently soft, thin, and open, cervical ripening techniques are employed. This may involve the use of a mechanical method such as the Foley catheter or a balloon induction. A small tube is inserted into the cervix and filled with fluid to apply pressure, facilitating softening and thinning. In some cases, a medicinal method involves the insertion of hormonal pessaries containing prostaglandin during a vaginal examination to soften the cervix.
- **Breaking of Waters/Rupture of Membranes:** If the cervix has started to dilate and thin, breaking the amniotic sac may be considered. A sterile instrument called an amnihook is inserted into the cervix to rupture the membranes, allowing the amniotic fluid to drain. This action encourages the baby's head to press down on the cervix, stimulating contractions.
- **Syntocinon Administration:** If cervical ripening and membrane rupture alone do not initiate labour, the synthetic version of the hormone oxytocin (syntocinon) may be administered intravenously. Syntocinon mimics the body's natural hormone that triggers labour. Dosage is carefully regulated to ensure effective contractions without excessive intensity.
- **Monitoring and Support:** Throughout the induction process, continuous monitoring occurs for the mother and baby. This assesses the progress of labour, the baby's well-being, and the mother's vital signs.

ROSIE & MOLLY

Hypnobirthing had always been a path I aspired to explore, a choice I envisioned if ever blessed with pregnancy. Limited to brief readings and conversations with a few friends who had embraced its techniques, I yearned to delve deeper, eager to put it to the test for my own impending births. Given my profound fascination with the birthing process, it felt like the natural and right direction to take.

I received a recommendation to contact Lynsey, and from that moment, I felt assured it was the correct decision. Lynsey effortlessly instilled a sense of calm, enabling us to shift our focus towards the impending arrival of our beautiful baby. Embracing the positives, letting go of worry, and allowing our bodies to follow their innate course became our newfound approach.

Engaging in 1:1 sessions, my partner and I were able to sit down as a couple, preparing for what felt like the best birthday party ever – the birth of our child. Lynsey empowered us to assert our right to question decisions and make informed choices when deemed necessary. She addressed our queries, guided us through potential scenarios, and outlined the various options available at each stage.

At 40+4, after careful consideration, we opted for induction due to concerns about the baby's growth. Despite warnings, including from my midwife, about the potential duration of induction, I was determined otherwise. To our delight, after a mere 5 hours of labour, our beautiful Rosie made her entrance, and we found ourselves on cloud 9. Becoming a mother exceeded all expectations, and the desire to relive the experience led us to welcome our second bundle of joy, Molly, 2 years and 6 days later.

With the guidance of Lynsey's refresher course, along with her unwavering support, I experienced a natural labour this time, devoid of pain relief and lasting just 5 hours once again. The empowerment derived from this natural birthing experience was immense, yet the willingness to opt for induction if necessary persisted.

In the midst of pregnancy's cacophony of advice and negativity, Lynsey stood as the beacon of wisdom. An absolute gem with an abundance of knowledge, she holds a special place in our hearts, and her influence on our birthing experiences is truly cherished.

ESMEE

I can honestly say that I had the most incredible labour and birth experience, exceeding all my hopes and expectations. When faced with the decision of induction at 12 days overdue, I was able to make an informed choice. Opting for induction with the pessary, I had my first one at 5 pm, followed by another at 11 pm. Strong contractions ensued, and remarkably, by 3:30 am, I had reached 7 cm dilation.

Subsequently, I was transferred to the midwifery suite, where the ambiance was transformed for my comfort. The midwife, creating a serene atmosphere, turned off all lights except a star projector, played soothing wave sounds, and even set up a fan. During contractions, I focused on my place of perfect peace, imagining myself on my paddleboard in the sea. It was a mental anchor that helped me navigate through the intensity.

By 5:30 am, the baby's heart rate fluctuated significantly, prompting us to decide to exit the pool for closer monitoring. Attempting different positions, I eventually found comfort on my back. Although the midwife set up the pool again, it proved challenging to pick up the baby's heart rate. Facing the possibility of an episiotomy, I resisted, opting to try a bit longer. Fuelled by a bottle of lucozade and a burst of determination, I pushed fiercely, and at 6:55 am, her head emerged, followed by the rest of her.

The euphoria of feeling her come out and having my baby girl placed on my chest is a moment etched in my memory. This profoundly positive experience, I believe, was shaped by the knowledge gained through your birth education and hypnobirthing techniques. I am genuinely eager to embrace the birthing process again with anticipation and confidence.

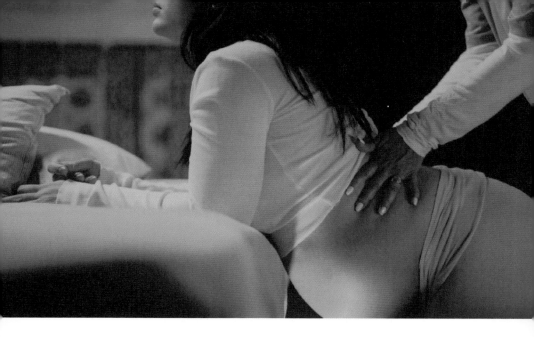

HOME BIRTH

Home birth can be an excellent choice for a birthing setting because it provides a familiar and safe environment. Usually attended by two midwives, either from a home birth team or community midwives, ensuring dedicated care for both the mother and the baby.

The National Institute for Health and Care Excellence (NICE), after reviewing evidence in the United Kingdom, concluded that home birth is as safe as hospital birth or a midwife-led unit for low-risk second and subsequent births, with some outcomes being even better. However, for first-time pregnancies, there is a slight increase in risk compared to a birth in a midwife-led unit.

Home birth is an ideal option for individuals who have:

- · An uncomplicated pregnancy.
- · A singleton pregnancy (one baby).
- · The baby in a head-down position (cephalic).
- · Labour initiating spontaneously between 37 and 42 weeks of gestation.
- · Ultimately, the decision regarding birth location is yours to make.

If you opt for a home birth, the midwife will be on-call for your delivery, usually from 38-42 weeks of gestation, but specifics may vary. The home birth team will provide necessary equipment before the on-call period, including pain relief options and essential items such as waste disposal, baby weighing scales, sterile gloves, and suturing equipment.

While most home birth teams do not supply birthing balls, comfort aids, or birthing pools, discussing and organising these items yourself is crucial.

Contrary to a common misconception about home birth, you have access to pain relief options, including gas and air (entonox) and stronger options like pethidine or Diamorphine, except for an epidural.

Being at home allows you to utilise various comfort aids, such as hot baths, showers, TENS machines, and Hypnobirthing breathing techniques.

Advantages of home birth include:

- Feeling more relaxed and in control in your own environment.
- Avoiding the interruption of labour by transferring to a hospital.
- Lower likelihood of needing interventions like assisted delivery (forceps or ventouse) compared to a hospital birth.
- Increased chances of having a midwife you have built a rapport with during labour.
- No need for separation from your partner after birth, as there are no visiting hours in your own home.
- The ability to get into your own bed after birth and have the food you desire.

Considerations for a home birth:

- Situations may arise during home birth that recommend transferring to a hospital.
- These situations include bleeding from the vagina not considered a normal show, high blood pressure development, signs of distress in the baby, the need for stronger pain relief, labour slowing or stalling, suboptimal positioning of the baby, evidence of meconium in the waters (indicating distress), and incomplete detachment or retention of the placenta.

ANGUS

My husband and I opted for Lynsey's refresher course in preparation for the birth of our second baby. The course served as a comprehensive reminder of all the hypnobirthing techniques that proved immensely helpful during our first birthing experience. Additionally, it covered the biomechanics of birth, providing us with valuable insights.

Feeling positive about our second birth, we decided to transfer to the home birth team around the halfway mark. Lynsey had equipped us with the necessary tools to strive for a calm and relaxed birth within the comfort of our own home.

As Lynsey emphasises, each birth is unique, and this certainly held true for us. Our first child was born 13 days past the estimated due date, and the first stage of labour was remarkably fast. In contrast, with our second child, labour commenced a day after the due date, but the initial stage was prolonged due to his back-to-back position (of which I was unaware).

The hypnobirthing techniques, particularly the breathing, relaxation, and massage, proved invaluable during the extended first stage. Managing with just these techniques and later incorporating the TENS machine, I reached out to Lynsey at one point due to concerns about the prolonged duration. She expertly calmed me down and even recorded an additional relaxation track for me, aptly naming it the 'time to come out, baby' script

Although my contractions were irregular and not closely spaced due to the back-to-back position, they intensified significantly. Prompted by my husband's suggestion – particularly when I began making cow noises – I called maternity assessment. A home birth midwife arrived, examined me, and confirmed I was fully dilated with the baby almost in the correct position. The birthing pool, prepared promptly by my husband, provided relief for my back discomfort. Employing the breathing techniques, along with some gas and air towards the end, facilitated a beautiful, calm birth. Angus was born in the pool, creating a magical experience.

Without Lynsey's course, we would never have had the confidence to attempt a home birth. Our gratitude towards her for enabling two such positive birthing experiences knows no bounds. To all expectant parents, I wholeheartedly recommend Lynsey's course. It transformed my apprehension about childbirth, and for that, we sincerely thank you, Lynsey!

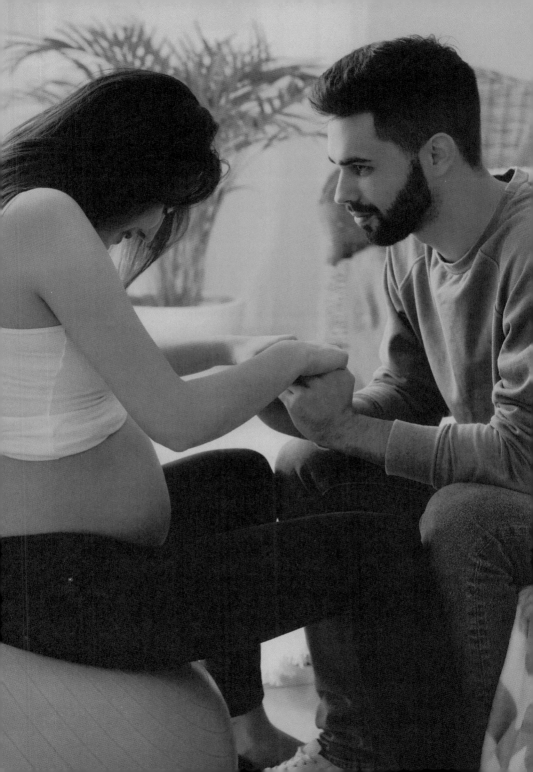

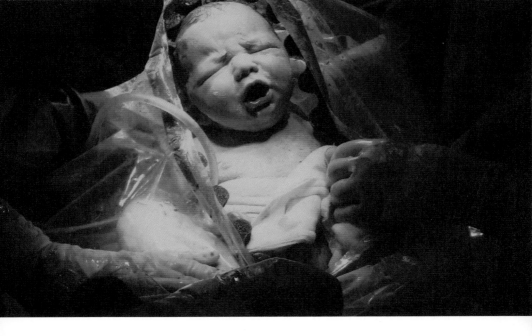

CESAREAN SECTION

A Cesarean section, also known as C-section, is a surgical procedure utilised for delivering a baby by making an incision in the mother's abdomen and uterus. While generally considered safe, this procedure comes with associated risks and benefits, with different options available based on specific circumstances. Let's delve into these aspects in greater detail.

Risks of C-Section:

1. **Infection:** Similar to any surgical procedure, there is a risk of infection at the incision site or within the uterus.
2. **Blood loss:** C-sections may involve more blood loss compared to vaginal deliveries, potentially necessitating blood transfusions in some cases.
3. **Injury to organs:** There is a small risk of accidental damage to organs, such as the bladder or intestines, during the surgery.
4. **Blood clots:** Immobility following a C-section increases the risk of developing blood clots in the legs or lungs.

5. **Longer recovery time:** Recovery after a C-section typically takes longer compared to a vaginal birth, accompanied by discomfort and pain during the healing process.
6. **Increased risk for future pregnancies:** Although the risk is very low, C-sections may slightly elevate the risk of complications in subsequent pregnancies, such as placenta previa or uterine rupture.

Benefits of a C-Section:

1. **Planned delivery:** C-sections can be scheduled in advance, allowing for better preparation and coordination with healthcare providers.
2. **Emergency situations:** C-sections can be life-saving when complications arise during labour, such as fetal distress, umbilical cord prolapse, or placental abruption.
3. **Reduced risk of birth injuries:** C-sections may lower the risk of birth injuries, such as shoulder dystocia, particularly in cases where the baby is significantly larger than average.
4. **Control over timing:** C-sections can be performed on specific dates, offering flexibility for medical or personal reasons.

Options related to C-section:

1. **Planned C-section:** A prearranged surgical delivery, often scheduled before the onset of labour or for specific medical reasons.
2. **Emergency C-section:** An unplanned procedure performed when complications arise during labour, endangering the health of the mother or baby.
3. **Gentle or family-centred C-section:** This approach aims to create a more positive birth experience by involving the parents in the delivery process, allowing for immediate skin-to-skin contact and breastfeeding soon after birth if possible.

JONAH

Upon discovering my pregnancy, the excitement of experiencing the journey overwhelmed me, especially after a previous miscarriage just three months earlier. A reassurance scan brought immense relief as I witnessed the flickering heartbeat, reassuring me that this time everything would be okay. I was aware of the impact stress can have on the body and developing babies, so I committed to becoming a relaxation expert for both myself and my growing baby.

Listening to my hypnobirthing relaxation became a daily ritual, providing a quick escape from stress, except for occasional interruptions by my husband's snoring during our relaxation sessions. The harmonious connection between my relaxation and the delightful movements of my baby reinforced the positive impact.

As we discovered the baby's gender, the anticipation of becoming a family of three intensified. Approaching the end of my pregnancy, the eagerness to experience labour and apply my practiced techniques grew. Witnessing the transformation in my husband, armed with hypnobirthing skills, was equally amazing. His role as my birthing partner became clear, even if I suspect I might have requested more massages than necessary.

The due date came and went, prompting an informed choice for induction due to the baby's size. Once in labour, skepticism lingered despite my hypnobirthing knowledge, but the techniques proved invaluable. Bouncing on a birthing ball, listening to relaxation, and dancing to the Carpenters and Dirty Dancing soundtrack created a serene atmosphere.

Transitioning to the labour ward, I continued to move around with supportive midwives. Despite the suggestion of rupturing my membranes, I maintained control, dancing and singing through contractions. Opting for an epidural later, the breathing techniques kept me calm, and the room's atmosphere remained relaxed and fun.

With the arrival of day staff, a familiar midwife, Tracey, brought calmness and reassurance. Despite the unexpected deviation from my initial birth plan, Tracey's support, along with Stuart's, brought me back to focus. The empowerment to choose a cesarean section when needed was profound, and the birth of our son, Jonah, on June 30, 2014, marked the culmination of a uniquely empowering and positive birthing experience. Though the planned pool birth didn't materialise, the right birth unfolded, leaving me eagerly anticipating the prospect of doing it again.

ORAN

For as long as I can remember, childbirth petrified me. I was never sure where that fear stemmed from—perhaps torturing myself with too many episodes of "One Born Every Minute," or the fact that, in society, a dramatic birth story is all people seem to want to tell, and it's what is portrayed in the media.

Once I met Ross, I knew I absolutely wanted to have a squad of children with him, but I always wondered how I'd actually get to that point with this fear hanging over me. The answer came after a few too many wines, which all became very real very soon, and that's when we met Lynsey!

I'd never heard about hypnobirthing until I fell pregnant, and another mum mentioned to me that she had done it. So, I started to research amidst my sheer panic, and Lynsey's name consistently came up as the person to go to. I booked Lynsey's private 1-1 course, where she came to our house over a period of four weeks.

Lynsey taught us so much that we had no clue about; it surprised me how little I knew.

We learned a huge amount—too much to list—but a few key learnings were how the body works in labour (my husband loved this bit as it was scientific!), how the mind works, our options and choices, relaxation techniques, and what to expect in labour, hospital, and after birth. Most importantly, from the above, we learned it was our birth, and we had a lot of choices to make.

I had decided early on that I wanted a c-section but was unsure how to approach this, as I wasn't aware you could request one without any medical grounds (another learning from Lynsey!). Lynsey helped me overcome my nerves about "asking" for one and prepared me for any questions I might be asked by medical professionals, but I never got many, and my planned c-section was booked for a week before my due date.

In the weeks running up to my due date, I expected to have a total wobble and go into a state of anxiety, but it didn't happen. I listened to Lynsey's podcasts every night and read about positive birth stories as advised. Even the night before my c-section, I managed to sleep, which I couldn't believe!

On the day Oran was born, everything went exactly how I'd really wanted. I was calm, informed, and extremely excited. We were fourth on the list for the day and spent the hours waiting in the theatre bay just chatting about how excited we were, counting down the moments until it was our turn to go. The surgeon and anaesthetist both came to meet us in the bay to introduce themselves and spoke us through the procedure (although we already knew what to expect, as Lynsey had gone through this with us). My calmness was accelerated when I found out my friend's husband was going to be the anaesthetist at our birth! Soon it was finally our turn! There's no doubt the theatre is a bit daunting when you first arrive, but everyone was so friendly and warm, chatting away. Once I had my spinal (something else I had been worried about, but this wasn't sore at all!), Ross was allowed in, and everyone got to work. Nothing was painful; I knew exactly what was happening. Lynsey was in my ear on my podcast, everyone continued to chat away, Ross was smiling with our midwife, and within minutes, baby Oran arrived squealing her lungs out—the most reassuring sound in the world! We were back through to recovery within 30 minutes, into the postnatal ward within a few hours, and home the next afternoon.

As I said to Lynsey in a text when Oran was born, the whole birth (and recovery!) has been an absolute dream, and I'd do it a hundred times over.

We'll never forget how Lynsey helped us make this all possible.

ARCHIE

Like many people, I struggled with low self-esteem, anxiety, and an innate fear of anything medical, especially considering I had never been in a hospital. The combination of these factors seemed particularly daunting during pregnancy and, of course, labour. The potential for fear to overwhelm me and taint my birth experience was a concern, and I knew I needed to regain control and shift the balance. I didn't want my baby to meet his mum for the first time when all she could feel was nervousness and fear.

This is where hypnobirthing with Lynsey came into play...

I chose to have a membrane sweep on my Estimated Due Date (EDD) due to concerns about my baby measuring "big" (3.7kg at 38 weeks). Although I had a mostly healthy pregnancy and wasn't medicated for it, intermittent problems with raised blood pressure prompted the decision to nudge me towards a vaginal delivery. Hypnobirthing played a crucial role in helping me make this decision, making it feel very much like my choice.

After the sweep on Thursday (fairly pain-free), I felt exhausted and unwell around 30 hours later. I messaged Lynsey, and ten minutes after sending the message, my waters broke—an experience I wanted, and the timing was perfect. Unfortunately, the color of my waters indicated potential issues, but I remained remarkably calm. I showered quickly, focusing on my place of peace under the blossom tree in Pollok Park, a spot I revisited mentally throughout labour.

Bags packed, husband prepared, I made a calm call to maternity assessment. They confirmed my waters had broken, but the baby had passed meconium, posing infection risks for both baby and me.

Given the infection risk, leisurely birthing wasn't an option. I agreed to a hormone drip and received antibiotics intravenously. Despite a lifelong fear of needles, I stayed calm and positive, focusing on meeting my son. Difficulties finding a vein during the six attempts to fit a cannula didn't shake my composure.

Throughout the evening and night, strong contractions ensued, and as planned, I delayed pain medication, using breathing techniques and meditation. Confirmed sepsis and feeling unwell led me to opt for gas and air, eventually moving to diamorphine. The possibility of an emergency c-section loomed if no progress was made by 2 pm. I remained unfazed and focused on delivering vaginally. By 2 o'clock, no progress, and I accepted that meeting my son was imminent.

Wheelchair offered, but I chose to walk to the theatre, bantering with surgeons about my scar's location and remaining calm during a successful spinal. Even in theatre, I was in a place of peace, and an hour later, 18 hours after entering the hospital, Archie was born, a healthy 8lb 7.

In recovery, significant blood loss occurred, but my mindset and approach throughout the labour experience, a beautiful and positive one, were all thanks to hypnobirthing with Lynsey. Conversations with midwives, doctors, calm moments with closed eyes, the sound of rain, Christmas songs, or my husband's gentle breathing—all contributed to a lovely experience. The low lights, quiet and peaceful atmosphere, and the overwhelming feelings of excitement and love made it truly beautiful. Grateful to Lynsey, Mark and I have a beautiful son who met his Mum and Dad when all they felt was love and excitement. Thank you, Lynsey!

SOFIA

Discovering my pregnancy was a thrilling and unexpected surprise, especially since we had been informed that IVF was our sole option for conception. The desire for a perfect pregnancy and birth arose, leading me to initially choose a home birth for its perceived calmness, reduced intervention, and gentle introduction of the baby into the world. Enrolling in Lynsey's hypnobirthing course equipped me with knowledge about our remarkable bodies, meditation practices, and breathing techniques that fostered a serene delivery, along with strategies for my husband's supportive involvement. I felt prepared and calm about birthing our baby.

However, my pregnancy encountered challenges, including sickness until 36 weeks, swelling, fatigue, and the development of Gestational Diabetes. Due to the latter, I was advised against a home birth, and with the baby "measuring big," options of an elective C-section or induction before the due date were presented.

Facing the choices of waiting for a natural arrival, induction, or elective C-section, I employed the BRAIN technique to list pros and cons based on our circumstances. Although a home birth was no longer feasible, the hypnobirthing course enabled us to make an informed decision without succumbing to fear. While a twinge of disappointment lingered, opting for an elective C-section felt right for us at that moment.

The hypnobirthing techniques continued to be valuable, and I persisted in listening to tracks and planning the day before and the morning of the C-section. The night before, we cherished our last meal as a couple, sent the dog for a sleepover, and enjoyed a cosy evening in.

The morning was relaxed and exhilarating, akin to embarking on a luxurious holiday. Arriving at the hospital early, there was no room for parking debates, and an unusual tranquility enveloped my husband and me. The supportive staff contributed to an overwhelming sense of calm as we proceeded to the theatre for the momentous occasion.

Being needle-phobic, the cannula posed the biggest challenge, but employing hypnobirthing breathing techniques enabled me to endure it with minimal fuss. Throughout the epidural process, I remained in my own bubble, serene amid the commotion around me. The experience felt like an intimate moment with my husband as Sofia was delivered and placed in my arms. Time seemed to stand still, and the background faded away until we returned to the ward, cocooned in our serene bubble.

In the end, there is no definitive or flawless method for a baby to enter the world; there exists no "perfect" birth. Effective decision-making based on prevailing circumstances is within one's control, and hypnobirthing equips you with a toolkit to navigate this process adeptly. Opting for a C-section was the right choice for us, resulting in a calm, gentle, and beautiful introduction of Sofia into the world.

KATIE

We had an incredibly positive experience with our planned section, and the difference we both felt before, during, and (most notably for me) after has been indescribable. We are now much more relaxed, at peace, and confident about the entire situation.

On the morning of the planned section, I had a delightful time getting showered and organising the kids for school. I then took Robbie to school, returning home to spend the remaining time playing with Maggie and cherishing those precious moments with them before our eagerly anticipated change. We arrived at the hospital at 11 am, following instructions. Due to other sections being more complicated and various issues, we were the very last name on the list, being the only easy and straightforward case of the day. However, we were content with this, as it meant John and I had plenty of time just the two of us. We utilised this time chatting, laughing, relaxing, and watching movies. Thankfully, we had a laptop and headphones, which came in handy as there were some less than respectful families in our vicinity, but that didn't impact our experience. Eventually, we were the last two left in our room, and the quiet and peaceful atmosphere was truly lovely. We had visits from the anaesthetist and the surgeon, both of whom were incredibly supportive of our requests for a gentle section and skin-to-skin contact.

As it was our turn to go down to the theatre, nerves kicked in, but the "3,2,1 relax" technique proved to be a lifesaver. I had instructed John to say this to me if I started getting stressed, and it instantly reset my mind to calm. John chose not to come into the theatre while I received the spinal, as he isn't comfortable with such procedures. He waited outside, and I used my breathing techniques and "3,2,1 relax" to stay calm. Experiencing the spinal while being so lucid was different and not pleasant, but it did not detract from the overall experience. Walking into the theatre and having everyone say hi and introduce themselves was also quite surreal.

Once all the anaesthetic was administered, John was brought in, and the anaesthetist engaged us in conversation, asking about the kids. This made the surgery progress without me realising it had started (John watched the entire process in the reflection of the lights). Before I knew it, the surgeon was instructing to drop the drape, and John helped me raise my head to see Katie's little head emerging. The surgeon joked with me, assisted in delivering Katie's shoulders, body, and legs with gentle pushes on my stomach, which I didn't even notice. After 60 seconds of delayed cord clamping just at my wound, Katie's cord was cut, and she was brought straight to me, placed against my face. She was briefly taken away for checks and a nappy, then returned to me, put on my chest with one of my hands holding her and one of John's hands keeping her still and safe. She stayed there throughout the time I was being stitched up, an experience that felt both timeless and fleeting.

When it was time to leave the theatre, John was given Katie, who was wrapped up to keep warm while they moved me. Once settled, she was given straight back to me for skin-to-skin contact, and we were both covered up to maintain warmth. The entire experience was incredible and everything I could have hoped for.

So far, Katie is the most settled and content little person. Her big brother and big sister are absolutely enamored with her, and our love for her knows no bounds. We are immensely grateful for the help and guidance you provided us with Maggie's pregnancy and birth, as well as with Katie's. It was a total game-changer.

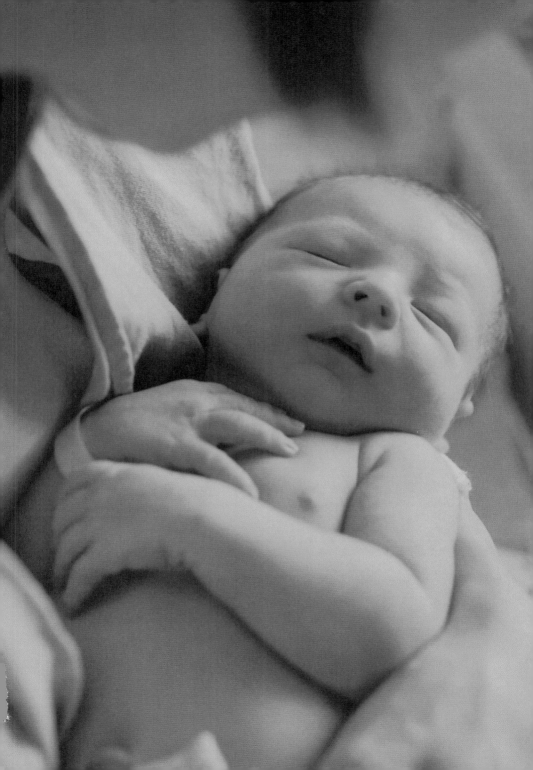

CONCLUSION

Each birth story encapsulates the extraordinary journey of bringing new life into the world. These narratives are not merely tales of labour and delivery; they are testament to the strength, resilience, and sheer marvel of the birthing process. Every birth is unique, an intricate tapestry woven with the threads of individual experiences, emotions, and circumstances.

Through these inspiring stories, the aim was to foster confidence in the innate ability of the human body to bring forth life. By sharing diverse accounts, we celebrate the ways in which women navigate the transformative journey of childbirth. There's a resounding message echoing through these pages – the absence of a universally defined "right" birth. What matters most is the birth that aligns with you and your baby, a deeply personal and intimate experience that only you can discern.

Your birth journey is a profound chapter in your life, and the birth of your baby marks not an ending, but a magnificent beginning. Remember, your birth matters, and within each story lies the profound realisation that birth, in all its forms, is an awe-inspiring and miraculous event.

So, embrace the diversity of these stories, find solace in shared experiences, and relish the fact that the journey is uniquely yours.

Birth, Actually... is amazing.

Elevate your birth experience with the empowering courses I offer at Born This Way Hypnobirthing.

Discover more about our transformative options:

- Explore our courses at **bornthiswayhypnobirthing.com**
- Private **one-to-one sessions** are available both in-person and via online, ensuring personalised support for clients near and far.
- Join our **group Hypnobirthing classes** held around central Scotland fostering a community of shared knowledge and encouragement.
- For flexibility, consider our **on-demand digital course** – a video-based program designed for you to navigate at your own pace.